STRENGTH BALL TRAINING

Third Edition

Lorne Goldenberg

Peter Twist

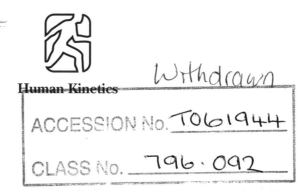

Human Kinetics

Library of Congress Cataloging-in-Publication Data

Names: Goldenberg, Lorne, 1962- | Twist, Peter, 1963-
Title: Strength ball training / Lorne Goldenberg, Peter Twist.
Description: Third Edition. | Champaign, IL : Human Kinetics, [2016] |
  Includes bibliographical references.
Identifiers: LCCN 2015048809 | ISBN 9781492511540 (print)
Subjects: LCSH: Weight training. | Exercise. | Balls (Sporting goods)
Classification: LCC GV484 .G65 2016 | DDC 613.7/13--dc23 LC record available at http://lccn.loc.
gov/2015048809

ISBN: 978-1-4925-1154-0 (print)

This publication is written and published to provide accurate and authoritative information relevant to the subject matter presented. It is published and sold with the understanding that the author and publisher are not engaged in rendering legal, medical, or other professional services by reason of their authorship or publication of this work. If medical or other expert assistance is required, the services of a competent professional person should be sought.

The web addresses cited in this text were current as of February 2016, unless otherwise noted.

Acquisitions Editor: Michelle Maloney; **Developmental Editor:** Anne Hall; **Senior Managing Editor:** Elizabeth Evans; **Copyeditor:** Jan Feeney; **Graphic Designer:** Denise Lowry; **Cover Designer:** Keith Blomberg; **Photograph (cover):** Rick Etkin; **Photographs (interior):** Brenda Williams and Rick Etkin; **Visual Production Assistant:** Joyce Brumfield; **Photo Production Manager:** Jason Allen; **Art Manager:** Kelly Hendren; **Associate Art Manager:** Alan L. Wilborn; **Illustrations:** © Human Kinetics; **Printer:** Versa Press

We thank Dean Nuels of Twist Sport Conditioning Centre in Vancouver, British Columbia, for assistance in providing the location for the photo shoot for this book.

Human Kinetics books are available at special discounts for bulk purchase. Special editions or book excerpts can also be created to specification. For details, contact the Special Sales Manager at Human Kinetics.

The video contents of this product are licensed for private home use and traditional, face-to-face classroom instruction only. For public performance licensing, please contact a sales representative at **www.HumanKinetics. com/SalesRepresentatives**.

Printed in the United States of America   10   9   8   7   6   5   4   3   2   1

The paper in this book is certified under a sustainable forestry program.

Human Kinetics
Website: www.HumanKinetics.com

United States: Human Kinetics, P.O. Box 5076, Champaign, IL 61825-5076
800-747-4457
e-mail: info@hkusa.com

Canada: Human Kinetics, 475 Devonshire Road Unit 100, Windsor, ON N8Y 2L5
800-465-7301 (in Canada only)
e-mail: info@hkcanada.com

Europe: Human Kinetics, 107 Bradford Road, Stanningley, Leeds LS28 6AT, United Kingdom
+44 (0) 113 255 5665
e-mail: hk@hkeurope.com

Australia: Human Kinetics, 57A Price Avenue, Lower Mitcham, South Australia 5062
08 8372 0999
e-mail: info@hkaustralia.com

New Zealand: Human Kinetics, P.O. Box 80, Mitcham Shopping Centre, South Australia 5062
0800 222 062
e-mail: info@hknewzealand.com

E6572

STRENGTH
BALL
TRAINING

Third Edition

CONTENTS

EXERCISE FINDER

Exercise	Stability ball	Medicine ball	Additional equipment	Video	Page number
Core Stabilization					
Balance Push-Up	✔				66
Bridge Ball Hug	✔				58
Bridge Perturbation	✔		BOSU DSL stability ball	▶	84
Bridge T Fall-Off	✔				52
Bridge With Medicine Ball Drops	✔	✔		▶	56
Closed Kinetic Chain (CKC) Ball Hold	✔				62
Dual-Ball Survival Rollout	✔			▶	75
Full-Body Multijoint Medicine Ball Pass		✔		▶	82
Jackknife	✔				46
Kneeling Ball Self-Pass and Tracking	✔	✔			59
Kneeling Hold and Clock	✔			▶	72
Kneeling Medicine Ball Catch	✔	✔			76
Kneeling Rollout	✔				80
Lateral-Jump Ball Hold	✔			▶	64
McGill Side Raise With Static Hip Adduction	✔			▶	49
Medicine Ball Single-Leg Balance Left to Right		✔		▶	96
One-Leg Opposite-Arm Medicine Ball Pass		✔			94
Progressive Tabletop	✔				78
Prone Balance	✔				48
Prone Balance Hip Opener	✔				50
Reverse Balance Push-Up	✔			▶	68
Seated Humpty Dumpty	✔	✔			74
Squat to Supine to Sit-Up			BOSU DSL stability ball	▶	88
Stability Ball Static Lateral Crunch With Medicine Ball Punch-Out	✔	✔			90
Standing Bar Twist With Medicine Ball Squeeze		✔	Loaded weight bar		60
Step and Push Back		✔			92
Supine Bridge Ball Hold	✔	✔			86

Exercise	Stability ball	Medicine ball	Additional equipment	Video	Page number
Core Stabilization (*continued*)					
Supine Stabilizer Scissors	✔			▶	54
Up Up, Down Down	✔			▶	70
Core Rotation					
Alternating Open-Step Medicine Ball Lunge With Long-Lever Rotation		✔			118
Back-to-Back Stop-and-Go		✔		▶	117
Goldy's Static Lateral Helicopter	✔			▶	110
Medicine Ball Standing Twist Against Wall		✔		▶	123
Medicine Ball Split Russian Twist		✔			120
Over-the-Shoulder Throw		✔			102
Prone Twist	✔				108
Russian Twist	✔				98
Side-to-Side Rotation Pass		✔			112
Standing Overhead Medicine Ball Rotation		✔			116
Standing Rotary Repeat			BOSU DSL stability ball	▶	122
Strength Ball Prone Thoracic Rotation	✔		Dumbbell		114
Supine Bridge With Cross-Body Pass	✔	✔		▶	100
Supine Rotator Scissors	✔			▶	106
Twister		✔			104
Legs and Hips					
Alternating Stability Ball Hip Extension With Single-Leg Eccentric Knee Flexion	✔				132
Goldy's Leg Blaster	✔		Cable		148
Hip Extension and Knee Flexion	✔			▶	126
Hip Power Initiation	✔			▶	150
Knee Tuck			BOSU DSL stability ball		128
Kneeling Side Pass		✔			162
Lateral Squat With Ball Push		✔			164
Lateral Wall Squat	✔				131

(*continued*)

Exercise Finder *(continued)*

Exercise	Stability ball	Medicine ball	Additional equipment	Video	Page number
Legs and Hips *(continued)*					
Leg–Hip–Core Multidirectional Control	✔				168
Lunge to Press and Track		✔		▶	158
Lunge With Medicine Ball Pass		✔		▶	154
O'Brien Hip Extension With Static Hip Flexion	✔				144
Plyometric Medicine Ball Box Jump		✔	Plyometric box		138
Poor Man's Glute Ham Raise Rollout	✔			▶	130
Prone Ball Hold With Knee Drive	✔				152
Repeated Dual-Foot Long Jump		✔			135
Reverse Lunge and Rotate		✔			156
Single-Leg Rotations	✔			▶	160
Single-Leg Squat			BOSU DSL stability ball	▶	146
Single-Leg Stride Squat		✔			140
Squat Press			BOSU DSL stability ball Dumbbells		166
Stability Ball Side-Supported Hip Extension	✔				136
Stability Ball Split Squat With Dumbbell	✔		Dumbbell		134
Wall Squat	✔				142
Chest					
Ball Walk-Around	✔				186
Dip With Medicine Ball or Stability Ball Squeeze	✔	✔			192
Dual-Ball Fly	✔				176
Incline Dumbbell Press	✔		Dumbbells		170
Jump-Out to Push-Up	✔			▶	180
Jump Push-Up	✔			▶	182
Medicine Ball Chest Pass		✔			188
One-Arm Dumbbell Press	✔		Dumbbells		200
Push-Up Pass		✔			198
Standing–Lying Partner Push-Up and Press	✔			▶	201
Standing Medicine Ball Press-Away		✔		▶	184

Exercise	Stability ball	Medicine ball	Additional equipment	Video	Page number
Chest (*continued*)					
Standing Partner Stability Ball Chest Press	✔				190
Strength Ball Decline Dumbbell Press	✔		Dumbbells		194
Supine Chest Push to Self-Catch	✔	✔			196
Supine Dumbbell Press and Fly	✔		Dumbbells	▶	174
Supine Push and Drive	✔		Dumbbells	▶	172
Walk-Out to Push-Up	✔			▶	178
Shoulders and Upper Back					
Cross-Body Rear Delt Raise	✔		Dumbbells		206
Isodynamic Rear Delt Raise	✔		Dumbbells		210
Medicine Ball Athletic-Ready Unilateral Wall Press		✔			224
Medicine Ball Push Press		✔			220
Medicine Ball Shoulder-to-Shoulder Pass		✔		▶	230
Medicine Ball Squat-Away Posterior Chain Wall Hold		✔			226
Prone Front Raise Lateral Fly	✔		Dumbbells	▶	214
Prone Medicine Ball Transfer		✔			222
Prone Row External Rotation	✔		Dumbbells		204
Pullover	✔		Dumbbells		212
Reverse Tubing Fly	✔		Slastix tubing with handles	▶	208
Scapular Pull	✔		Dumbbells		228
Scapular Push-Up	✔			▶	232
Seated Rotator Cuff Pull	✔		Slastix tubing with handles		218
Supine Lat Pull and Delt Raise	✔		Dumbbells	▶	211
Supine Pull-Up	✔		Power rack with barbell	▶	216
Abdominals, Lower Back, and Glutes					
Abdominal Side Crunch	✔				254
Adam's Medicine Ball Ab Lockout		✔		▶	236

(continued)

Exercise Finder *(continued)*

Exercise	Stability ball	Medicine ball	Additional equipment	Video	Page number
Abdominals, Lower Back, and Glutes *(continued)*					
Back Extension	✔				246
Ball Sit-Up to Medicine Ball Pass	✔	✔		▶	255
Barbell Hip Extension With Medicine Ball Squeeze		✔	Barbell		248
Hanging Knee Raise With Medicine Ball		✔	Pull-up bar		252
Reverse Back Extension	✔		Flat bench	▶	244
Stability Ball Reverse Rollout	✔		Power rack and bar		250
Supine Lower-Abdominal Cable Curl	✔		Cable with ankle strap	▶	238
Supine Lower-Abdominal Curl and Crunch	✔			▶	240
V-Sit Medicine Ball Transfer		✔			242
Wrap Sit-Up	✔				234
Biceps, Triceps, and Forearms					
Eccentric Accentuated Biceps Curl	✔		Dumbbells	▶	258
Incline Triceps Extension	✔		Dumbbells		260
Medicine Ball Push-Up		✔			266
Medicine Ball Quick Drop and Catch		✔			272
Medicine Ball Walk-Over	✔			▶	268
Overhead Medicine Ball Wall Bounce		✔			262
Triceps Blaster	✔			▶	264
Wrist Curl and Extension	✔		Cable or dumbbells		270
Whole Body					
Angle Lunge With Horizontal Medicine Ball Rotation		✔		▶	284
Ax Chop With Hip Flexion		✔		▶	294
Medicine Ball Circuit		✔			302
Medicine Ball Overhead Jump and Throw		✔			298
Medicine Ball Overhead Lateral Bounce to Floor		✔			296
Medicine Ball Romanian Deadlift to Hip Flexion		✔			290

ACCESSING THE ONLINE VIDEO

This book includes access to online video that includes 53 clips demonstrating the complete exercise programs. Throughout the book, exercises marked with this play button icon indicate where the content is enhanced by online video clips. ▶

Take the following steps to access the video. If you need help at any point in the process, you can contact us by clicking on the Technical Support link under Customer Service on the right side of the screen.

1. Visit www.HumanKinetics.com/StrengthBallTraining.

2. Click on the **View online video** link next to the book cover.

3. You will be directed to the screen in figure 1. Click the **Sign In** link on the left or top of the page. If you do not have an account with Human Kinetics, you will be prompted to create one.

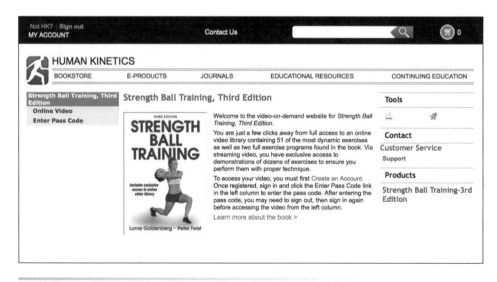

Figure 1

4. If the online video does not appear in the list on the left of the page, click the **Enter Pass Code** option in that list. Enter the pass code that is printed here, including all hyphens. Click the **Submit** button to unlock the online video. After you have entered this pass code the first time,

you will never have to enter it again. For future visits, all you need to do is sign in to the book's website and follow the link that appears in the left menu.

Pass code for online video: GOLDENBERG-9X2-OV

5. Once you have signed into the site and entered the pass code, select **Online Video** from the list on the left side of the screen. You'll then see an Online Video page with information about the video, as shown in figure 2. You can go straight to the accompanying videos for each topic by clicking on the blue links at the bottom of the page.

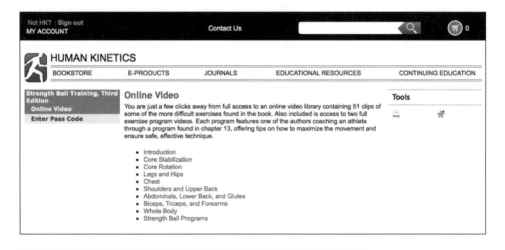

Figure 2

6. You are now able to view video for the topic you selected on the previous screen, as well as others that accompany this product. Across the top of the page, you will see a set of buttons that correspond to the topics in the text that have accompanying video:

Core Stabilization	Abdominals, Lower Back, and Glutes
Core Rotation	Biceps, Triceps, and Forearms
Legs and Hips	Whole Body
Chest	Strength Ball Programs
Shoulders and Upper Back	

7. Once you click on a topic, a player will appear. In the player, the clips for that topic will appear vertically along the right side. Select the video you would like to watch and view it in the main player window. You can use the buttons at the bottom of the main player window to view the video full screen, to turn captioning on and off, and to pause, fast-forward, or reverse the clip.

INTRODUCTION

From the very first edition of *Strength Ball Training,* we have endeavored to create a resource based on sound biomechanical and physiological parameters. The world of exercise science is ever evolving, and with that as with any exercise technique, there continues to be research that may either support or play down the effectiveness of any particular exercise tool or method. Since 2007 there has been a number of research papers in support and against the use of the strength ball as an optimal means of training.

We have always believed and promoted the use of our exercises and progressions as a tool in our toolkit, not a be all and end all solution to your fitness needs. By integrating the ball and our exercises you will certainly see improvements in your strength, spinal stability, mobility, and your ability to move in a more efficient manner.

We have updated the science section of *Strength Ball Training* to touch on new areas such as training the myofascial lines, our real body armor; how using the strength ball can impact your sports performance if you are an athlete; or how you look and feel if you just want to be lean and fit. In this edition we demonstrate how it can help you repair a body from injury and restore it from disuse. Read on and see why we do what we do with the ball!

Since the publication of the first edition of *Strength Ball Training,* there has been a significant increase in the use of stability balls and medicine balls in fitness programs. Participants reacted favorably to the natural athletic feel of strength ball training, which is different from the mechanical nature of muscle isolation techniques. The integration of whole-body strength training with core, balance, and coordination training spawned an audience of trainers, coaches, and participants asking for more. Our response is *Strength Ball Training, Third Edition.*

Training with strength balls has had an immense impact on the fitness industry. Personal trainers needed specialized education to coach whole-body coordination and advance their teaching skills beyond what was required for selectorized weight machines. Training became more portable, allowing exercise specialists to take clients outdoors. Coaches could bring exercises right into their sport environment—on the court, on the field, or at the rink. Retailers noticed increased demand for these products. Where else can you find an exercise device you can use in your home that can give you thousands of variations of exercises without the need for a huge, expensive line of equipment?

To appreciate the power of strength ball training, you must only understand that your body functions as a unit, with muscles firing sequentially to produce the desired movement. Some muscles contract to produce movement, others contract to balance the body, and others contract to stabilize the spine and hold it in a safe position. Other muscles kick in each time your body recognizes a shift in position or to correct an error, such as a loss of balance. Your body is a linked system that coordinates athletic actions. Throwing a football requires the leg, torso, and upper-body muscles to work together and contract in the correct sequence. Your body functions as a linked system in everyday life as well, such as when bending over to pick up a baby and lifting the baby overhead to produce a smile. This movement is dependent on leg, torso, and upper-body strength—both prime movers and stabilizing muscles. This is the foundation for what we present in the third edition of *Strength Ball Training*.

Over the years, we have improved our strength programs by adding multi-joint, full-body exercises with free weights that incorporate the entire body, dumbbell lifts while standing on one leg, and medicine ball drills to activate the entire body. However, the most versatile tool has proved to be the stability ball. Strength training with a stability ball offers an exciting breakthrough. The opportunity to make the body function as a unit to execute an exercise has tremendous utility in sport performance, adult functional fitness, kids' training, injury rehabilitation, and fitness for aging populations. Most important, you train with an unstable (round) surface. Strength and balance are summoned in unstable and unpredictable environments—such as when slipping on icy stairs, lunging to catch a falling child, and withstanding a check to continue running while catching a lacrosse ball. These real-life conditions require contributions from all muscle groups. Each joint and muscle senses position in space and changes to other linked joints and muscles to react and produce the appropriate action. This linked system is a kinetic chain that produces functional movement safely.

The stability ball exercises in this book integrate instability into the closed kinetic chain through prone and supine positions that build from the center of the body to the periphery. Medicine ball drills add a dynamic load that requires full-body, coordinated actions. Catching a weighted ball outside your midline trains the deceleration and responsiveness properties of muscles, placing emphasis on the core and posterior chain. Together these tools produce improvements that support athletic movements (such as skiing down a mountain) and full-body everyday activities (such as digging in a garden), which keep the muscles and joints healthy and reduce the risk of injury. It is really about training and integrating the body as a whole and taking the focus away from development of only the muscles you can see in the mirror.

Stability balls and medicine balls are making a positive contribution to the sport rehabilitation, athletic conditioning, and general fitness fields. However, as with all exercise, well-executed technique produces optimal results, while poor technique at best produces nothing and at worst causes injury. Although balancing and moving on a ball or catching and throwing a weighted ball seem like simple and playful concepts, activating your body's proprioceptive mechanisms and challenging your low back and deep abdominal stabilizers are serious undertakings. Since primary goals include improvement of posture, movement mechanics, and athletic skill, an illustrative book demonstrating effective exercises and proper technique is long overdue. In this book you will find the answers to your questions. To enhance the third edition, we have included access to full exercise program videos. Each program features one of the authors coaching an athlete through a program found in chapter 13, offering tips on how to maximize the movement and ensure safe, effective technique. You can repeat the programs as many times as you like to fit the length of time you have for your workout.

Coaches, trainers, therapists, and self-guided fitness enthusiasts alike can follow the exercise progressions and modifications in the book and videos to customize each exercise for their level. It is important to know simple modifications for each exercise to make them easier or harder. When you first begin, you will most likely need to simplify certain exercises so they require a little less strength or coordination to make them appropriate to your level, to produce results, and to stay safe and injury free. You also improve with training, so eventually you will need to know how to change an exercise to make it more challenging and to require more strength and coordination.

The bottom line in real life and sport is that you are only as strong as your weakest link. For most people this is core, or torso, strength. How many people do you know with low-back pain? How many athletes have experienced abdominal, hip flexor, and groin strains? Strong legs and strong arms along with a weak core are an injury in the waiting. Strength ball training builds from the core out to the periphery, accommodating your upper and lower body while turning your core into your strength. A stronger core is your speed center and strength center. Most movements are initiated and supported with the core muscles, and this is not just your superficial six-pack muscles. It also includes more important muscles deep in the abdominal wall that protect your spine and stabilize movement. The demand of swinging a golf club is a perfect example. A golf swing is mostly core, a little legs, and even less upper body.

You will note the importance of building strength that is transferable to sport and everyday activities. It is safe to say that in the sporting world, golfers require the lowest amount of fitness of most athletes. A high percentage of golfers lack the core strength to be their best. Most have experienced back pain. If they work out, many rely on floor-based sit-ups, stationary bikes, and selectorized weight machines that isolate specific muscles. Ironically, golfers use high-velocity rotation in a standing position 70 to 100 times per round. In addition to the high-velocity rotations, golfers load only one side of the body by swinging the club in one direction, which contributes to many of the problems they have as they become injured. Golfers need excellent core stability and strength in the legs and hips for powerful rotation. You need to choose an exercise style that will prepare you for the specific task to be performed.

While many other sports use rotation for skill execution—throwing and kicking a ball, swinging a racket—they also need smart and reactive muscles for agility, balance, quick direction changes, body contact, falling, jumping, bounding, and many other athletic attributes. For athletes, the goal of strength ball training is to teach the body to move more skillfully. For functional fitness, incorporating whole-body stability and balance into an exercise increases the metabolic costs, causing you to expend many more calories as you build strength.

In 2002 when the first edition of *Strength Ball Training* came out, we used the general research pertaining to balance and the nervous system to justify the use of training we had long known to be beneficial. There were few documented studies at that time to justify the use of stability and medicine balls in training programs. It seems that research is constantly lagging behind the practical coaching of today's leading exercise practitioners. Forward-thinking strength and conditioning coaches are constantly finding methods and tools to take their clients and athletes to a higher level, sometimes to the chagrin of the researchers. There was a coach who said that if he had to wait for those with PhDs to justify with documented studies what he was doing in the training room, he would have to wait almost a full Olympic cycle before his methods were validated by science, rather than by the gold medals his athletes were winning.

Many traditional practitioners are skeptical of anything beyond an Olympic bar and a dumbbell. Some scientists are locked into periodization paradigms borrowed from Eastern bloc countries in the 1950s, defensive of any advancement that does not align with the model in which they have invested their career. We recommend being confident in one's knowledge yet also humble, because it is a fluid process in which we always strive to find new methods to generate better real-life results. This statement is more of a commentary on a progressive period of exercise development rather than a negative view of research. As the authors of *Strength Ball Training,* we both come from a background in science. As an exercise physiologist and conditioning coaches, we have lived in the academic research world and continue to be active in research today. We have been prudent in designing exercises that are founded on solid scientific principles, anatomy, neurophysiology, and biomechanics. But it is noteworthy that our pace of developing new methods of training is faster than the ability of science to validate the utility.

Since 2002 several researchers have had an opportunity to catch up to the practitioners and test some of the training methods and products. Some interesting research validates the use of stability balls in training programs, which you can find in chapters 1, 2, and 3 of this book. You can also read about requisite stable strength exercises you should be able to complete before progressing to many of the unstable drills presented in this edition of *Strength Ball Training.* We present advice on selecting appropriate equipment as well as the general rules about making each exercise more or less difficult. Within each specific exercise are recommendations you can follow, including progressions (such as adding weight, decreasing the base of support, or increasing the speed of movement). We think these guidelines will add value to your program, help you enjoy the exercises, and produce the best results.

The online video reinforces the written and pictorial instructions from the book for some of the more difficult exercises. Within the exercise chapters you will notice a video symbol on certain exercise pages. This is an indication of which exercises are included in the online video. We have also provided video for two of the routines in chapter 13.

Best of all, strength ball exercises are fun to do because of the constant challenge. It is not only about lifting more weight. It is also about having fun exploring how to coordinate more complex exercise variations. As you become more experienced with the exercises as we present them to you, you will find there are endless variations that could easily triple the size of this book. The constant challenge will motivate you to adhere to your program, and athletes and fitness participants will respond very positively. Take advantage of this powerful tool and get to the core of the matter with *Strength Ball Training!*

CHAPTER 1

THE STRENGTH BALL ADVANTAGE

Strength ball training involves fitness and sport workouts using both stability balls and medicine balls. The instability of a stability ball and the dynamic property of a medicine ball are tools used in practicing the most modern functional training methods.

The practice of integrating a ball with human motion dates to the second century AD. Today's stability ball was developed in the early 1960s as a toy for children. It was adopted by physiotherapists as a means of improving patients' proprioception and balance (Posner-Mayer 1995). Recognizing that several physiological mechanisms receive positive results from stability ball training, strength and conditioning professionals and personal trainers adopted stability balls in their exercise programs.

Stability ball and medicine ball exercises require all parts of the body to communicate and work together, from toe to fingertip, so the entire body understands how to share demands and contribute to the task at hand, second by second, through any activity. Your body is an amazing machine, with many sensory capabilities that allow it to carry out proper motor function. These sensory capabilities all fall under the term *proprioception.*

Proprioception

Proprioception involves the sensation of joint movement and joint position feeding information to the brain so the body's "software" can compute what physical actions are required. In this way it contributes to the motor programming for neuromuscular control required for precise movements and contributes to muscle reflex, providing dynamic joint stability (McGill 2015). Mobility and stability are two attributes that give you freedom of motion when you need to move into position and strength during walking and running or when you need to brake before changing direction. Strength programs that transfer results from the gym to life and sport develop stability and improve mobility. Excellent proprioceptive capabilities are evident when an athlete absorbs a hit on the ice or playing field and maintains balance as a result of the firing of the required muscles at the optimal time, in the correct order, with an appropriate level of force. For this to occur, several physiological events occur inside the muscle. Receptors are all over the body—in the skin, tendons, joints, and muscles—and will react when they sense a change to the tissue and to the entire body position as a whole, detecting forces, pressure, vibration, motion, speed, joint angles, and instability. These changes are computed by the central nervous system and, after the brain decides how to react, the proper signals are sent to the muscles via the spinal cord and nerves for muscle contraction and hence movement.

Stability occurs when the brain commands muscles to contract across joints, creating muscle stiffness, which stabilizes joints with the appropriate strength at the appropriate time so you can load motion. For example, to live independently, an elderly person must stabilize the pelvis and knee joints on each foot strike while walking down stairs and contract muscles at the right time. To move freely while playing sports, you need full range of motion in the joints, and muscles of the core, hips, glutes, and legs need to fire and contract on each foot strike. This is true during a casual run, and the demands are magnified during abrupt changes in direction, such as during on-court footwork required for winning a tennis rally.

Fine Points of Myofascial Performance

The reactive stability required in agility patterns during sudden stops and changes of direction not only is key to functioning and performance but also greatly affects appearance. Of course you can see that strength training builds muscle. But not all strength training improves movement capabilities. Because the ebb and flow of stability and mobility permit human motion, the more you train with strength balls, the more confident and capable your physical movement becomes.

The energy costs of handling a medicine ball and managing a stability ball are much higher than with traditional exercise; as a result, strength ball training expends many more calories than traditional training does. Improved stability and mobility give you a body that simply works better in motion. Improved physicality enables you to participate in activities involving greater physical exertion, which burns more body fat and elevates your fitness.

Application of Strength to Stability

Let's look deeper at the clever software that orchestrates the body's hard drive. The application of strength to stability is so important that specific muscles of the body have more sensory capabilities than others. The rotator and intertransversarii muscles, for example, are very small segmental muscles in the spine. (See figure 1.1.) They cannot produce a high level of

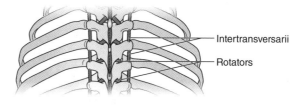

Intertransversarii

Rotators

Figure 1.1 Rotator and intertransversarii muscles.

force but are very efficient at sensing vertebral position because they have an abundance of muscle spindles. Muscle spindles are sensitive to length and rate of stretch and will cause a muscle contraction when their threshold is reached.

The rotator and intertransversarii muscles, because of their minimal cross-sectional area, act as position transducers for each lumbar joint to enable the motor control system to control overall lumbar posture and avoid injury (McGill 2015). This is important in the spine and other articular structures during extreme ranges of motion because these muscles and neighboring ligaments provide neurological feedback that directly mediates reflex stabilization in the muscles around the joint (Lephart et al. 1997). For instance, all the segmental muscles must contract to help stabilize the spine during movement. This movement may be the result of performing something consciously, or it may be unconscious as the result of a hit on the playing field or a sudden change in terrain while running trails. As you will learn, strength ball training will enhance your body's unconscious reactions that produce appropriate movement, which often means the difference between regaining control and suffering a sport injury.

Muscle Fibers

Muscle spindles are the mechanisms that mediate the response from plyometric exercise. As the main stretch receptor in the muscles, when it is stretched at a particular rate and length, the muscle spindle will detect the change, send a signal to the spinal cord, and receive a message directly back that will initiate a reflex contraction in the muscle, resulting in a powerful concentric muscle contraction (Chu 2013). This is known as the myotatic stretch reflex. Here's how it works: Your extrafusal (EF) muscle fibers contract or elongate to produce movement. You also have intrafusal (IF) muscle fibers that run parallel to the EF fibers, where they are well positioned to report on the magnitude and rate of muscle lengthening and tension. (See figure 1.2.) When the EF fibers quickly elongate, the IF fibers stretch along with them and send a message to the spinal cord to inhibit the agonist and powerfully contract the stretched muscle. It produces this result with an extremely quick turnaround time because the message travels directly to the spinal cord and back without having to take the longer journey up to the brain.

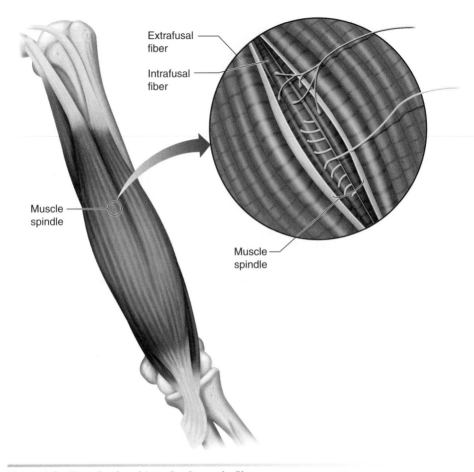

Extrafusal fiber

Intrafusal fiber

Muscle spindle

Muscle spindle

Figure 1.2 Extrafusal and intrafusal muscle fibers.

Connective Fibers

Golgi tendon organs (GTOs) are another type of receptor in the body. More specifically, they are in the musculotendinous junction. The GTOs are attached end to end with extrafusal muscle fibers so they can monitor and respond to tension in a muscle and its tendon. If GTOs reach their threshold, they will send an inhibitory signal that will result in the muscle's relaxing and shutting down. This is a protective mechanism that the body uses under very heavy loads. A novice weightlifter, for example, would have a very low threshold, because his body has not fully adapted to the intramuscular and neuromuscular benefits of weight training. An advanced lifter, through proper training, would have a much higher threshold than his novice counterpart, allowing him to lift much heavier loads.

Nerve Fibers

Skin receptors can enhance the deeper receptors located in the muscle. Receptors in the skin of the wrist and fingers can provide information on wrist and finger movements. Visual and auditory sensors also play a part in the body's ability to function. The ability to see an oncoming hit or to hear a warning cue from a teammate allows the body to prepare itself for action. This may be in the form of muscle contraction and body segment stabilization for a change in direction to absorb the hit efficiently or make the play. A hockey player moving the puck down the ice while his head is down is vulnerable to a crushing open-ice hit. As his teammate yells, "Heads up," he will instinctively tense up, look around, and prepare his body for a hit.

Information Pathways

All information described previously is translated for the central nervous system (CNS) by many receptors. The coordinated efforts of all these mechanisms allow the body to meet the challenge of functional movement in an unpredictable, changing environment.

The receptors detect change to the body and send their signals via afferent pathways to the CNS. There it is broken down and sent to a motor control center, where a decision will be made regarding the mechanism of muscle contraction. The resulting muscle contraction comes about through efferent motor pathways, which is like your computer software operating the hard drive. There, neural information is transformed into physical energy. This whole mechanism is a complex scientific phenomenon beyond the scope of this book; however, a cursory understanding helps you appreciate the value of strength ball training and know what to emphasize during exercise execution. Figure 1.3 illustrates

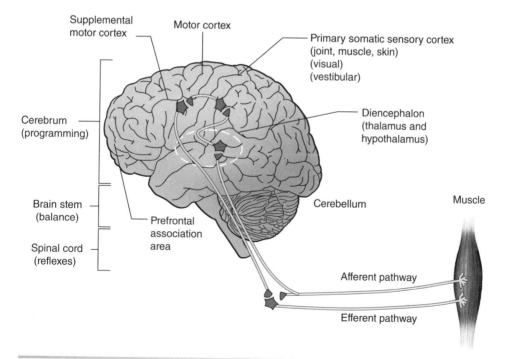

Figure 1.3 Functions of the central nervous system.

information pathways while the rest of the book guides you in performing exercises to maximally exploit the sensors and receptors that tell muscles to work harder, so they get stronger and your entire body becomes smarter during human motion.

Myofascial Lines: Your Body Armor

In strength ball training are many foundational knowns leading to an understanding of the body as a human system. From there you learn how to define what you impose on the body—the vision to unlock the potential of this amazing anatomy in motion. After identifying the why and determining how it is overloaded, the how is exercise guidelines that dictate the movement and load during each drill so you can achieve adaptations.

The long fascial lines that run up and down the body add greatly to the why of strength ball training. The body is designed to share information and collaborate on function, which strength ball training overloads for maximum gains.

One pathway discussed earlier involves nerves carrying sensory data through the body to the muscles, flooding your software with information about your body's positioning and motion and the environment you must act in and computing commands to the muscles at a rate of up to 170 miles per hour. It does not peak there. Fascial tissue communicates at 700 miles per hour. Fascia is one interconnected network of sensor-rich tissue around all cell structures serving in part as a protective sac but more impactfully to training outcomes, playing a role in stability, mobility, force, and communication.

Your myofascial tissue runs in long head-to-toe and hand-to-hand lines, all interconnected together to make up one map of larger-functioning continuities that wind longitudinally and spirally through the body. As the largest and richest sensory organ in the body, with 9 times as many sensory nerve endings as muscle, the transmission speed (700 mph) and volume of nerve endings (9 times more than muscle) make for a massive and constant communication system related to internal tension and force. With ongoing messaging between fascia and muscles, you use information from your fascial lines to determine the position of your body in space and perfect the synergy with muscle toward desired motor outcomes. Strength ball exercises that produce length in the body under load and instability feature specific design elements to grab the fascial systems' full attention.

Muscle and fascia interface, affecting function, strength, stability, and communication along the fascial lines. Continuous in long lines, fascia talks to the next muscle up or down the body line. Because the fascial sinew that envelopes muscles communicates across attachment points, muscles do not actually have to cross a joint to affect mechanical movement. The biceps, for example, is one element in a continuous fascial plane that runs from the outside of the thumb to the fourth rib and beyond.

An ebb and flow exist between muscle and fascia. When muscles become compromised, exceeding their capabilities to hold loads in certain mechanical positions in particular when at a biomechanical disadvantage (which happens often in sport), the web of myofascial tissue contributes more. Fascia can be tensional for stability but also contributes to mobility and movement. The structure of the fascial matrix linking muscles creates a massive weave of muscle tissue capable of force and power generation. This accelerates the view of a more global approach to the human system as opposed to individual parts of a machine that are trained separately then fit together like assembling parts on a machine. In fact, whole groups of muscles are linked by fascia; therefore, discovering the synergies between muscle and fascia helps you understand how the body can—and should—move and how it can be challenged and loaded to exploit this synergistic relationship and varied roles of fascia.

Training the fascial lines sends energy into the whole human system, unifying the body. From the field of neurogenesis you can understand that what fires together wires together. In strength ball training, exercises set up body angles, levers (arm length from midline), and lines of pull—the resistance you exert against perpendicular to the body or at variable angles to the prime movers. Together, this formula asks the fascial system to contribute more, which leads to a strong body armor of fascial tissue and muscles. Whole-body strength and fitness are enhanced by loading motion in specific ways so there is a significant neural connect to the fascial planes, which reboots your computer with more functional and reactive programming.

Repairing Injuries, Restoring Bodies

Strength ball training is an effective way to awaken the body and mind, make muscles more alert, and activate maximal muscle activity from head to toe. Addressing deficiencies in the neuromuscular systems, as described previously, has been a goal of therapists for many years. Lephart and colleagues (1997) believe that training to enhance joint muscle receptors should be used early in a rehabilitation protocol. Activities should focus on small yet sudden alterations in joint positioning that necessitate reflex neuromuscular control. Additionally, some researchers have discovered that there appears to be a better recruitment pattern when the focus on training initially is one of instability and balance followed by heavier-load strength training. This is even more apparent for women in terms of the role of the abdominal muscles and stabilization immediately after childbirth. Postpartum, it would take the abdominal muscles about 4 to 6 weeks to reverse the length changes and for motor control to reorganize. For example, the rectus abdominis takes about 4 weeks postpartum to reshorten, and it takes about 8 weeks for pelvic stability to normalize. It would be expected that during this period there would be minimal spinal support and stabilization from the slack abdominal muscles and their fasciae (Lederman 2010). This could increase the likelihood of low back pain and demonstrate the need for progressive exercise to bring a post-partum woman back to effective core strength and stability so that daily tasks do not put her at risk for injury. Returning to workouts after sedentary phases can begin with stability balls alone followed by integration of weight-loaded exercise using medicine balls and heavier dumbbells and further progressing to explosive Olympic-style weightlifting if training for speed power sports.

Athlete and Nonathlete Treatments

To begin the initial sequencing, as previously stated, the progressions should be the introduction of unstable exercise combined with and followed by heavier strength training. From a recruitment standpoint, the activation of antagonists and synergistic muscles will enhance muscle activation (Anderson and Behm 2005). This can be achieved through balance and postural activities. We have implemented this with our injured athletes to help them recover their athleticism and to prevent reinjury when reentering their unpredictable read-and-react competitive environment. These types of exercises stimulate muscular coactivation (Lephart et al. 1997). This will allow for greater loading tasks for the specific joint, which will result in greater increases in strength, which will result in stronger and more functional joints. This phenomenon of increased balance and stability will lead to increased functional strength. Another progression that is successful is detailed in chapter 2: building from the middle of the body out to the periphery. The primary focus is on the preparation of the core out to the limbs. By performing specific strength moves for the core, in a variety of planes, using static and dynamic contractions, athletes see positive graduation to some of the more difficult unstable exercises and positive transfer to the playing field.

The concept of injuries and pain relates not only to athletes but also to the general population. One area that has been looked at from this perspective is pain during pregnancy. A woman who carries a baby to full term experiences a change in body structure, which can result in biomechanical issues with the spine and hips. A study by Yan and colleagues (2014) examined pregnant women who did not suffer back pain or had minimal pain during the period of 20 to 22 weeks of gestation while in a program using the stability ball. The women trained for 12 weeks, 3 times per week, for 25 to 30 minutes. The training group had significantly less low back pain and daily life interferences than the control group at 36 weeks of gestation. The authors concluded that including stability ball exercises during pregnancy may reduce low back pain during pregnancy and boost daily life functions.

Balance

Balance is a state of bodily equilibrium, otherwise known as the ability to maintain the center of body mass over the base of support without falling. Berg (1989) defines balance in three ways: the ability to maintain a position, the ability to voluntarily move, and the ability to react to a perturbation. All of these definitions are important for sport performance as well as for general human movement, which is challenged in balance tasks every day.

Muscles make up a continuous chain that attempts to overcome disturbances in the center of gravity. The chain begins in the ankle. When a challenge of balance forces the body to lean forward, the muscles in the back of the ankle, the gastrocnemius, will contract to counteract this movement to pull the body back in balance. If balance is forced backward, the anterior tibialis muscle will contract and work to pull the body back into the center of gravity.

While you stand on one leg, there is an increased challenge to balance from side to side, which will be counteracted by pronation and supination of the foot at the ankle joint. In some instances the sway of the body will be too great for only the ankle to counteract the balance challenge. When this occurs, the muscles in the legs, hips, and back counteract the movement. In this example of standing on one leg, breakdowns in strength and balance may be evident with lateral flexion (trunk), rotation (hips), poor posture (back), or excessive arm movement (shoulders and arms). The body will maintain or regain balance only if muscles act across all joints to hold the desired position.

Breakdowns are even more apparent in people who have suffered ACL injury. Postural balance can be significantly affected as a result of the loss of information supplied by mechanoreceptors in the knee joint. These receptors provide information about knee position and the movements of that joint. After an ACL injury, the neural feedback mechanism is hindered and the motor control of the knee is damaged, resulting in excessive movement in the joint and loss of postural balance. Post rehabilitation on a repaired ACL returns the individual to preinjury strength levels but also restores postural balance demonstrating again that body must be looked at from a fascial chain perspective.

Combined stability and balance play such a key role together, because they are the foundation of human movement. Stability and balance do not typically occur in isolation; rather, they work together to allow the body to move. The ability to maintain segmental control in the trunk contributes to spinal stability and reduces unnecessary movement between the vertebrae. This can decrease the risk of back pain by reducing tissue strain, deformation, compression, and overstretching. So the ability to keep a strong, stable, balanced body while at play or in daily activity will dictate overall ability to move effectively in any environment.

Remember that the body is a linked system. Each muscle has receptors to assess its relative position in space and the body's overall balance. They will communicate with each other, sharing information to produce the required movement, since they all have an equally vested interest in performing well and remaining injury free.

Research

In 2002 when the first edition of *Strength Ball Training* was released, there was limited research on the specific benefits of training with a ball and other unstable surfaces, such as wobble boards. Since 2002 there have been numerous papers written on this topic that support the notions we put forward in our first edition of *Strength Ball Training*.

One area that has received attention is the research on activation of the core musculature as well as how training the core with stable and unstable devices affects core recruitment. In a study from Memorial University in Newfoundland, Anderson and Behm (2005) looked at how unstable and unilateral (single arm or leg) resistance exercises affect trunk musculature. They used exercises that are commonly used in resistance training programs, such as shoulder press and chest press. They evaluated single-arm and dual-arm movements on an unstable ball and on a stable bench. They also used four exercises on a stability ball that challenged the core musculature in various planes and angles. What they found was something that many ball users have been experiencing for many years: Compared with exercises not involving the ball, instability exercises generated greater activation of the lower-abdominal stabilizer muscles (27.9 percent) with the core exercises and all core stabilizers (37.7 to 54.3 percent) with the chest press. Although there was no effect of instability on the shoulder press, the unilateral shoulder press produced greater activation of the back stabilizers, and the unilateral chest press resulted in higher activation of all trunk stabilizers when compared with bilateral presses.

Regardless of stability, the Superman exercise was the most effective trunk stabilizer exercise for activation of back stabilizers, whereas the McGill side bridge was the optimal exercise for lower-abdominal muscle activation. Anderson and Behm (2005) concluded that the most effective means for trunk strengthening should involve back or abdominal exercises with unstable bases. Furthermore, trunk strengthening can also occur when performing resistance exercises for the limbs if the exercises are performed unilaterally.

At the 2005 National Strength and Conditioning Association National Convention, an abstract research study by validated the benefit of using single-arm movements over bilateral arm movements and how they affected the core musculature. In comparing the bench press with the standing single-arm cable press, the authors discovered that the bench press provided greater activation of the pectoralis major and the erector spinae, but with the standing single-arm cable press the activation levels for the core musculature, including rectus abdominis and obliques, were double that produced by the standard bench press. They concluded that the bench press was better for hypertrophy and strength as a result of activation level, and the standing press was more optimal for core stability and torsional challenges and a more accurate representation of what happens to the core in a standing position. This is relevant to what we prescribe in this book, particularly regarding any movement that can be described as unilateral. For example, the one-arm dumbbell press and the balance push-up progression show how the core must work significantly harder when unilateral movement or balance is challenged.

Anderson and Behm (2005) concluded that the introduction of instability into an exercise increases the extent of muscle activation. But there is a cost, which appears to be force production. Although a person may not be able to exert a force at the same level as in a stable environment, there may still be benefits to be obtained by using unstable devices. The decreased balance associated with strength training on an unstable surface might force limb musculature to play a greater role in joint stability. One strong example involves a person squatting on a wobble board. During the squat, the EMG (electromyographic) levels were compared with those of a standard squat. The EMG levels for several core and leg muscles were significantly higher for the same submaximal load on the wobble board than on a stable surface. The authors believe that this may be attributed to their greater need for postural and stabilizing functions in the unstable condition. Since the first edition of *Strength Ball Training*, researchers have had time to conduct more studies in various academic fields to catch up with practitioners. The new research only urges us to pay even more attention to how muscle and fascia communicate and what they are designed to detect so we can more artfully put the body in positions with specific types of overloading that trigger the muscles to respond quickly and strongly to maximal improvement.

Over the last decade, stability ball training has become a vital tool for personal trainers and strength coaches. It has been controversial at times as researchers have attempted to discredit its use while many have supported it. This is inherent in any industry where a specific tool has shown great results. There will always be those with conflicting views and principles and alternative products and ideas. This is what generates interesting conversations, blog posts, and exchanges of ideas, which can easily be viewed on the Internet. We believe that the stability ball as *part* of a complete fitness program can have a positive impact on anyone who seeks safe options and progressions, and the research that has been completed to date supports this. There is no best in exercise science for everyone; there is only what you can do.

CHAPTER 2

TRAINING WITH THE STRENGTH BALL

Exercise has evolved and become so dynamic over the last decade that it has brought much innovation and excitement into the industry as a whole. Techniques that were once considered old, such as kettlebells and strength band training, are new again. With this as with any program, integration will be your key to the success in the most logical and fundamental ways. As you will see in this chapter, the concepts of progression, adaptation, and age-appropriate exercise are the main focus. The strength ball will provide you with an excellent workout on its own, but you will experience even further gains if you understand how to integrate these drills with other conventional weight training exercises.

Most strength training routines involve several exercises ranging from 6 to 10 movements. This will depend on the goal of the program, the phase of training you are in, and whether or not you are completing minicircuits in your workout. Our experience tells us that depending on your goal, you can do 20 to 40 percent of your exercises with a strength ball.

Positioning Strength Ball Training in a Workout

Strength ball training is useful for professional athletes, weekend warriors, or seniors seeking to enhance their strength foundation. Strength ball training can easily be adapted to meet a variety of needs and goals. Balls of various sizes and inflation densities as well as the weights and exercise variations used enable everyone to enjoy exercises appropriate for their skill levels. However, how, when, and how much these exercises are used can vary greatly depending on your goals and abilities. Strength ball training can define the complete workout for some participants, while in other applications it is common to integrate specific strength ball exercises with other types of exercises.

Dynamic Warm-Ups

The goal of a warm-up is not to stretch, and it is not just to warm a muscle. Traditional static stretches, which involve holding stationary poses, do little to prepare a body for action. In fact, current research indicates that preceding workouts and competitions with static stretching actually leads to lower strength outputs and slower speeds (Fradkin et al. 2010).

Dynamic warm-ups engage the mind and muscles in a way that makes muscles more compliant and responsive to the mind's commands in preparing the body to move. This mental focus sets up the muscles to be at their best for the rest of the workout, thereby optimizing your time in the gym for strength development.

Selecting less difficult strength ball exercises or using lighter loads is suitable for preexercise, prepractice, and pregame warm-ups. The low-impact, smooth weight-loaded activity takes muscles through dynamic ranges of motion, increases the temperature deep in the muscles to make them more pliable, and stimulates production of synovial fluid to lubricate joints. The instability promotes whole-body coordination, and the weighted medicine ball at the end of the body's levers activates both the muscles and the nervous system.

To begin your warm-up, you should choose an activity that will increase blood flow throughout the body, which will result in an increase in core temperature. This requires six to eight minutes of light cycling, jogging, skipping rope, or exercising on a cardio training machine such as a treadmill, elliptical trainer, or rowing machine. Once you complete the initial warm-up, progress to using some strength ball exercises for a more specific dynamic warm-up that progressively prepares the core musculature, legs, and arms for movement, balance, and force production.

Complete Functional Strength Workouts

Are you a general fitness participant looking for a bit of everything in your workout program? You can select exercises from each chapter to create a full-body workout stressing all parts of the body in roles of prime movers and stabilizers. To help get you started, we created the first one for you—a full-body strength program with aspects of mobility, flexibility, stability, balance, and reactivity—to help you achieve the physical function while strengthening the entire body. This approach significantly upgrades the workout experience if you're accustomed to exclusively using selectorized weight stack machines that require little thought, focus, or coordination. The challenge of recruiting the entire body to perform an exercise will help link the kinetic chain in order to develop smarter muscles that better communicate with the rest of the body. See chapter 13 for the stability and balance workout. Integrating balance and movement with strength is demanding both physically and neurally because it harnesses multiple muscle groups to heighten the metabolic cost, expending more calories.

We also recognize that many people prefer to use selectorized weight training machines, and for this reason we include a specific full-body reset program (chapter 13) to integrate with your machine-based workout, which will in turn bring about the benefits described in this chapter.

A complete functional strength workout incorporates the following elements. Training using stability balls and medicine balls, plus involving other tools such as dumbbells with the stability ball, facilitates exercise mechanics and coordination demands. Remember it is not the tool that determines the outcome. The tool accommodates certain exercises, yet it is you and how you decide to move through the exercise that determine your results. You might orchestrate motion more slowly to remove any momentum and keep tension on the muscles longer to up your strength outcomes while moving through your longest range of motion possible under load, netting more mobile joints via this effort. Training is an art—two people can do the same program, but one person might double the other's gains. To improve, be in control, stay present in the moment, and exercise with intent. Nowhere does this recommendation pay more dividends than when exercising with integrated instability.

As an adult exerciser, you would do well to alternate body parts, which allows you to progress through a sequence of exercises with minimal rest to sustain an elevated heart rate. Increasing exercise density is most effective when muscle groups are rotated in a way that permits top strength output in every set. Traditional circuit training tends to reduce the efficacy of each strength exercise to the point where fewer improvements are noticeable. We like to keep our adult clients moving but without compromising the quality of each exercise. Here is a sample rotation formula that permits best efforts in every set: alternating push and pull of legs, shoulders, and core; rest; and repeat. While this sustains high contributions from both the aerobic and anaerobic energy systems, you should engage in other aerobic activities, such as jogging or swimming, and integrate periods of anaerobic effort, such as hiking or cycling uphill.

Workouts for Young Athletes

When learning how to integrate strength ball training into an exercise program, you have various considerations. Not everyone is an adult exerciser. Young kids cannot be treated as miniature adults. All kids go through phases of growth and maturation, which require specific types of training. As kids age, they grow taller and then later add muscle mass. But before bones lengthen at a fast rate, their nervous systems develop. Prepubescent children (younger than 12 years) go through a phase of peak maturation of the nervous system. This is a stage in which their coordination, body awareness, and athleticism can be improved by training with complex exercises, during which they must solve the puzzle of coordinating each exercise. A great example is the squat movement. This is fundamental to all sports and general human movement, but children have a difficult time learning this simple natural movement. Children tend to round the back, knees drift too far forward, and they are unable to engage the hip extensors in a proper pattern. By using the strength ball wall squat, children can learn this pattern and reinforce proper body mechanics before moving on to the free-weight movement. Use the ball to establish the foundation and then layer on more neurally complex exercises, such as a reverse split lunge, with the trail foot or leg atop the ball. Advancing from the wall squat to a lunge (single-leg squat) position heightens strength and balance demands, recruiting more musculature up and down the body. A lunge introduces dual instability, so every muscle must contribute to the loaded motion.

Children aged 8 to 12 can complete one exercise for each body part and three or four core stability exercises to begin to build strength through interesting activity that improves their neural networks. Give younger kids (those below 8 years of age) minimal direction while turning three or four exercises into fun game challenges. Make sure the room is safe—the area is carpeted or padded and clear of clutter for safe exits from the ball's surface. Then just let the kids have fun and find their own way around the ball. Most home users and gyms have 65- or 55-centimeter balls. Prepubescent children fit better on a 45-centimeter ball that accommodates their height and allows them to use the ball constructively. Young children should avoid weighted medicine ball throws until they have the core and posterior chain strength to safely handle catches as well as the emotional maturity to pay attention to the structure needed when throwing and catching weighted balls.

Orient kids to the stability ball and avoid imposing too much structure. Lead them through the primal movements that their developing neural systems naturally crave, then allow their curiosity and interest in play to lead them to new exercise variations. Keep it fun and open-ended.

Balance and Physical Growth

Pubescent kids going through a peak skeletal growth phase, typically a period of awkward growth, can use strength ball training as a complete workout to help them become accustomed to their new height and weight and regain coordination. The low-impact nature of strength ball training frees kids from other high-impact training and activities that commonly cause injury during puberty when bone levers have elongated but muscles have not grown in length, size, and strength. A full-body general workout, performed at light loading, is a good place to start. Remember that training on the ball uses the *body mass* as the primary loading, then some exercises add tools like medicine balls, dumbbells, and tubing. Tall, lanky kids becoming accustomed to their longer bodies can modify exercises by keeping more of the body on the ball, which shortens the volume of body off the ball, decreasing load and increasing stability. In some exercises, they can also increase the base of support (feet or hands) where they need assistance coordinating proper exercise execution.

Naturally, since they are taller with longer legs, arms, and torso, but not yet bigger with strong muscles to support that frame, if they struggle too much with an exercise, simply omit it and select an easier option. Or find a more level appropriate way to execute the exercise. The best results are not from progressing exercises but rather often regressing them. When an exercise is regressed, it means meeting the clients where they are. In this way, they can perform the exercise better and hence work their bodies harder. Regressing something permits other things to be worked harder—properly. That produces the best improvements. Train smart.

Postpubescent kids go through a peak rate of muscular maturation once they have the circulating hormones needed for muscle hypertrophy, so it's a great time to capitalize on weight-loaded strength training. Using heavier loads or resistance at slower tempos through full ranges of motion creates the most muscle tension and stimulates adaptations in muscle growth. At this stage of growth and development, strength ball training should become part of their workout that includes lifting heavier free weights through multijoint actions.

Childhood Obesity

One special consideration is childhood obesity. It is a growing epidemic. There are many contributing factors: the quality of our food supply, convenience of fast food, sedentary entertainment, parental role modeling, family lifestyles, and economic constraints. Regardless, the fitness and health industries are too busy finding excuses and reasons why folks cannot achieve. We believe people can and are very passionate in our beliefs. Younger kids have access only to what parents avail. Healthy food is available around the perimeter of every grocery store. Avoid the aisles and feel great filling your cupboards and fridge with health and strength. Make activity a part of what the family does together. Parents get fit and show it is important to take care of themselves. Although "busy" is a badge of honor everyone waves in today's society, the reality is usually that folks spent dozens of hours each week watching television, playing video games, or surfing social media. Simply cut out TV. Exercise, pick up an activity, or play a sport. All three help kids spend more time around like-minded kids and make their interests contagious. Instill a positive mind-set around exercise, fitness, health, and food. It is not about calories, diets, and weight loss. It is about building a body that works, which is each person's personal vehicle. If your vehicle does not work well, it causes you to say no to opportunities to do things you enjoy, which literally shrinks your world, netting fewer experiences. When your body improves, it will take you more places so you can say yes to things you are passionate about and participate confidently in your physicality. More positive engagement in what you love naturally shifts your energy and attitudes, which you bring into your home and influence those closest to you with it—good attitude or negative attitude. Exercise, then, is about mind-set. The two are intimately linked.

Overweight kids need calorie-burning and health-promoting activity, but its focus should be on netting a more functional body that moves better navigating life's playing field. It must be a fun and positive experience or kids will be quickly turned off. Obese children often have less coordination and are more challenged by movement than healthy-weight, fit kids. Overweight kids can do better by using selectorized weight stack machines, the one activity in which they might outperform average-sized peers. Weight stack machines require little coordination, but they make strength development safer and more achievable for obese children. If the children have success, they might continue. After initial improvement, adding in simple strength ball exercises to improve their coordination and mobility will help them move more skillfully. Once they can move more skillfully, it is then possible to load up that more skillful movement, which is how we train athletes and active adults in our gyms. Strength ball exercises produce higher heart rates and activate more muscles than exercises without a ball, thus causing an expenditure of calories. Therefore, it helps people win the battle of calories in versus calories out. However, strength ball training requires much greater coordination and physical exertion than exercise without a ball, so take it one step at a time. We are here for anyone who desires to get better and ready to support anyone compelled to improve.

Sport Conditioning

The belief that you are in the weight room to build strength, not demonstrate it, is one that will go far in keeping you healthy and productive. On the other end of the spectrum are the athletes of all ages, the best of whom must perform and compete in organized chaos. The best in the world are true genetic anomalies. Absolutely anyone and everyone who is athletically inclined, all ability levels from recreational to professional, need to train all the pillars of sport performance: strength, speed, agility, power, and reaction time. The pillars of sport performance build on a foundation of functional strength. With a strong foundation, a developing athlete will realize more efficient gains in development when progressing to training more intense performance pillars. Think of the performance pillars as a diamond. The lower half shows what constitutes functional strength. Athletes begin here, improving their foundation, the platform on which the upper half of the diamond builds. So athletes may do a general functional strength workout and later progress into sport conditioning workouts. Function plus performance is when you see the most prolific displays of athleticism.

To maximize strength and explosive power and increase the size of muscles relative to the demands of their performance environment, athletes need to lift with heavy loads. Depending on training history, there could be some debate about when and how much heavy lifting is necessary. The use of heavy loads is a common practice for many athletes. In fact, one question you hear often in a strength training room filled with athletes is "How much can you squat or bench-press?" This kind of competitiveness promotes the use of heavy weights to improve performance in the bench press and squat, and it is probably one reason why so many overuse injuries occur in strength athletes. Yet training maximum strength is a characteristic that has been researched and proven to be a critical component of development when programmed appropriately.

Strength ball training is a very effective way to develop the functional foundation and improve how the body is unified and connected *before* heavy weightlifting commences. With that, the important point is that not only is maximum strength critical to performance, but balance and coordination also play a significant role. These two components are part of linked-system strength. This concept emphasizes how the body is linked together via fascia and connective tissue and how movements that are static, such as the bench press, provide very little carryover to sport performance and do not train the body's linked system. An exercise such as a single-arm dumbbell press on a stability ball would require the use of the pectoralis major (the prime mover) as well as all the core musculature to maintain a solid positioning on the ball. It also requires the use of the glutes and hamstrings so that the feet can maintain contact with the floor.

When we are in coaching mode with our athletes, we do not think about maximum strength in the classic sense (that is, bench press or squat). We recognize its importance, but we have the perspective of the body as a linked system. The components of linked-system strength as it relates to maximum strength can be enhanced through the use of the many strength ball drills in this book. Explore how you can define a prime mover such as push with the chest musculature while also integrated balance and movement so you train the whole body to eradicate any weak links and teach the body to practice firing the muscles in the correct order from the feet and ankles up the chain through to the fingertips where the prime movement is expressed. For example, a squat to a diagonal medicine ball push builds mobility and strength in the legs, hips, and low back; power is in the torso, chest, and shoulders, linking the body and summing power from ground up through to the hands. Using the body as a whole and firing muscles in the correct sequence help produce fluidity of movement.

As an athlete, you must also train speed, agility, quickness, whole-body reaction skills, and anaerobic capacity. Strength ball exercises for athletes are incorporated in an overall lifting program. Strength ball training is never the full program for elite athletes. We have shocked the industry's early violent opposition to balance training by having success generating hypertrophy (growth in muscle size) using instability as the training overload. Without question, to lift the heaviest weight when strength or power training, you should be up on your feet on a flat floor.

Strength ball training is more common in the lower half of the diamond where the foundation of function is enhanced and less common in the upper half of the diamond where programming is dominated by multidirectional running drills, plyometrics, and explosive lifting. Sport conditioning programs would, however, still involve a high volume of core stability exercises using stability balls and core rotation drills using medicine balls. Stability balls make up a small volume of the upper-body and leg exercises to complement athletic strength training with Olympic bars, dumbbells, and heavy medicine balls.

Bigger, Stronger, Smarter

If you're a bodybuilder or someone who strength trains recreationally with goals of increased muscle size and better appearance, you can use strength ball exercises to better connect the kinetic chain and improve communication of muscles and joints to perform better in heavy lifts. Strength ball training can help in pushing through strength plateaus by improving the neural pathways so you can use the software (brain and nervous system) as well as the hardware (bigger muscles) to drive your body to top performance.

If you use heavy strength training programs, you can use a strength ball exercise that integrates balance and secures high muscle activity to potentiate muscle right before a heavy, stable lift. You might also order a strength ball exercise immediately after a heavy stable lift to work on muscle coordination under fatigue. A set of unstable stability ball push-ups, for example, can activate the body to perform better in a flat traditional bench press. The key is to activate but not take it to fatigue.

Rehabilitation

Rehabilitating an injury is not just about letting nature do its job. Rest time is indeed needed for a muscle or ligament to repair. But along the way, a return to action is faster and more successful with less risk of reinjury through participation in a well-structured strength and movement program. An injured body can use strength ball exercises to rebuild damaged areas as well as recondition close-to-healed bodies so they return to action even better than before. Return-to-play exercises must be functional to ensure the injured area is ready to handle real-life action and sport action, not just walking and sitting.

Having a body that works, free of pain and full of abilities, is a true gift since the body is a vehicle and can limit your life experiences since the less your body works, the more things you are forced to say no to; the fuller your functional capabilities, the more you can say yes to. Greater participation in what you love to involve yourself in affects the vastness of your experiences and hence your learning and personal growth, knowledge, awareness, attitude, energy, and healthfulness. Society's lack of interest in the vehicle of the body is peculiar. Strength ball training will enable you to stand out from the crowd. By this point in the book, you have deeper understanding and motivation to train for function. This is best attacked proactively, but it is also an effective advantage after an injury.

If you are using rehabilitative exercises, you need to also re-educate your body to avoid a pattern of dysfunction, in which the body compensates to cover for an injury. For example, with an injury to the left knee, the right side of the body takes on more of the body mass. There is a short-term shifting of responsibility in the body, but this can cause problems in other areas of the body. Left unchecked, these new problem areas lead to further dysfunction and injury. The bottom line is that exercises must not only tackle the initial injury but also strive to tune up and attend to the rest of the body, which was also affected by the initial injury. The process of recovery from acute injury should be directed by a medical professional who is well versed in the mechanics of exercise. This is often not a doctor but a physiotherapist or athletic therapist. Be active in the communication—take your book to the medical professional to double-check what exercises can contribute to the process at that stage. The specialist may prompt you to focus on firing specific muscles during an exercise and make other meticulous adjustments that require professional guidance.

Initial injury is often caused by other problems in the body. We speak to treating the cause, not the symptom, and often an injury is caused by other weak links in the chain that, over time, cause a seemingly unrelated injury. If you have had an injury, chances are your body still needs to be corrected and you need to tune up what started the chain of events in your body that led to injury. Many people function with minor pain and strength imbalances that negatively affect their ability to perform at their best in activities and leave them at risk of further injury.

The process of re-educating the body need not wait for injury. Strength ball training at its best is proactive, activating your entire body as one linked system with high neural engagement to help you get better while *not* inured and keep you operating at your best.

Whole-body re-education includes smooth, whole-body strength exercises that fire muscles in the correct sequence and stimulate the proprioceptive system to repair software and muscles together. Strength ball exercises draw on multiple body parts to get the job done properly, forcing the body to work together and expose weak links in the kinetic chain. If strength ball exercise does not help correct patterns of dysfunction, try an easier version with the goal of laying a proper foundation in the body. If a weak link or any discomfort persists, refer to a medical professional who specializes in injury assessment and active, exercise-based rehabilitation. It is important for professionals such as personal trainers and coaches to stay within their scope of practice and refer clients to a team of professionals when their exercise protocols do not solve the problem. Chiropractors, physiotherapists, massage therapists, acupuncturists, naturopaths, and other specialists can benefit clients. Likewise, to link your exercise and sport goals to the process, you should select a sport performance coach and a medical professional who is competent and current in exercise application and knowledgeable about the demands of sport. If you are a home user, level-appropriate strength ball training will help build from the center of the body out and link the kinetic chain together. If you have a new injury or an old minor problem that persists, get the short-term advice of exercise and medical professionals who can give you hands-on assessment and map out your precise program.

Workouts During Travel

A deflated and folded stability ball is an excellent training tool to take on the road. It travels easily, and upon inflation it can be used in hotel rooms, at cottages, and in other locations. Many business people who travel frequently pack a ball and the *Strength Ball Training* book, using a hotel room for a quick and convenient workout. Strength ball training helps combat the fatigue of travel, helps reset the body's clock when changing time zones, and keeps you on a consistent schedule in your workouts. Given enough time, it is fairly easy to go for a short run or climb some hotel stairs for aerobic conditioning. Adding a whole-body strength ball routine keeps you progressing instead of falling behind on strength and function.

As single dads who run businesses and travel extensively to lecture and consult, we understand busy and stretched schedules. One of Twist's goals for his dozens of road trips each year is to return home feeling better than when he left. This requires a small amount of forethought: packing portable food, stopping for a quick grocery pickup after landing at the airport, and getting active each day no matter the time pressure. There is *no* better combat of mental fatigue or physical fatigue than neural-based exercise. A brief strength ball training workout that includes mobility and strength opens up the body, activates the body, and harnesses the movement-based instability to stimulate the brain.

Eating clean on the road is not difficult. It is a mind-set. If you are reserved to eating poorly, sleeping poorly and drinking too much on a road trip, you likely will. If you plan ahead with the intent to eat clean, drink a lot of water, and strength train for the duration of the trip, it all helps you get higher-quality sleep, and a successful road trip is often an achievable short-duration goal.

If you are a business traveler who does not feel safe running in an unfamiliar city, you can circuit through several strength ball exercises in your hotel room at a work rate that sustains an elevated heart rate to achieve fitness for the heart and lungs. This is accomplished by circuiting through lighter-load exercises without rest between sets to sustain a heart rate, effectively combining aerobic, anaerobic, and strength exercise into one portable workout.

Strength Ball Use in the Workplace

Most jobs have repetitive tasks, such as working on an assembly line or sitting at a desk typing and talking on the phone. Having access to strength balls allows for short active breaks to stretch and actively strengthen muscles and balance the body. A couple of short exercise breaks over the long term can improve strength, balance, and fitness. In the short term, an exercise break with an unstable ball activates all the muscles in the body, not just those used in the workplace, and recharges the body and mind. Taking a break from workplace tasks to awaken the mind and body can improve your work performance and prevent repetitive-use injuries. From a space allocation standpoint, many businesses do not have the resources to dedicate significant space to a fully equipped employee fitness facility. With a set of dumbbells or power blocks and a few strength balls, you can easily create a fully functional fitness room in a space as small as 225 square feet (~21 square meters).

Research now shows that even fit regular exercisers who sit all day for work may have a lower life expectancy. It is what you do hour by hour throughout the day that counts. If your work makes you a sitter, try active sitting on the ball at your desk. Or, better still, sit on your regular work chair to focus on your work at hand but take hourly microbreaks to mobilize and activate on the ball. That is a great place to brainstorm, solve problems, or reflect on business documents you need to make smart decisions on. The light exercise on the ball is also a stress reducer, which helps you think more clearly.

Choosing Exercises and Progressions

When starting any new fitness program, begin at a level that will reinforce proper technique and movement patterns. This is especially important with strength ball training, which also challenges stability. Once you have mastered a particular move, then you should continually challenge yourself with the appropriate exercise progressions to ensure progressive levels of success in your program.

Selecting Exercises

To get you started in your first full workout, include exercises from all chapters. Build from the center of the body out, preferentially training the core first and then the periphery (arms and legs). All of the exercises in this book stimulate good core activation, so an equal representation from all chapters works well because it ensures you check off all the prime movers and body parts to train the complete body.

To keep primary core exercise safe, work on abdominal and core stability exercises for several weeks as a foundation before training core rotation. Chest exercises using supine and prone positions are good examples of prime mover strength exercises that also build core stability with a neutral spine. Look for exercises that keep the hips square and aligned with the shoulders to build strength around the spine before progressing to exercises that rotate the torso or shift the hips' center of mass.

Preworkout Testing

The most accurate and individualized way to use strength ball training is to complete the battery of tests in chapter 3. These help you determine which muscle groups need most attention and your strengths and weaknesses. The focus is primarily on core strength and stability because this is the area that is most often injured or weak in more than 80 percent of people. Without a doubt, more intensive assessments are available to you, and you should certainly seek them out if you require them. These assessments can provide a more in-depth view of all joints and movements in your body. For example, someone may show evidence of high strength in prime movers (such as push, pull, legs) but lack stability and core control. Someone else may have high strength but poor mobility, while another may have low strength but excellent mobility. You should still begin by selecting an exercise from each chapter; however, the way in which you do the exercises is tailored to what the tests unveil as weaknesses. Restricted mobility? Use a fuller range of motion. Low strength? Use a slower tempo and wide base of support to achieve more time under tension and build greater strength. Low core control? Use a narrow base of support and select more primary abdominal exercises.

Remember that before even beginning strength ball training, and if you are new to strength training in general, you should develop some base-level strength with stability training, as described later in the section Precautions in this chapter. Once you are ready to begin strength ball training, note that the exercises in each chapter are listed in order from easiest to most difficult. This ranking is determined by the intensity of the physical exertion required as well as the complexity of the coordination needed for successful completion of the exercise. Skipping ahead will only cause your body to compensate and cheat to get an exercise done, setting you up for injury. Take your time and practice a group of exercises before progressing to new exercises of greater difficulty.

Keep in mind that within most exercises are tips on regressing to make an exercise easier and progressing an exercise to make it more challenging. Regressions are often applied on the spot, when you try an exercise and find it too difficult. A quick adjustment can make it more achievable. Progressions are often applied toward planning the next workout after you notice certain exercises have become easier to complete. Each workout should be a challenge to you. If you have achieved your repetition goal, you should consider a slight increase in your medicine ball weight, the addition of two or three repetitions per set, or an adjustment to the body mechanics to make the exercise more challenging. For example, during supine exercises, a longer torso off the ball and small base of support at the feet increase the requirement of muscle activation, strength, and control. Specific methods to increase the difficulty of an exercise are listed for each exercise. General rules for progressing an exercise are detailed in the following sections.

One of the most underused yet most effective ways to step-change progress is to regress something so you can progress something else. For example, increasing the width of the base of support is a regression that permits you to handle greater weight loading in a one-arm dumbbell supine press. The regression permits you to advance the loading and build more strength. In the same exercise, regressing the weight to a lighter load may permit you to adopt a single-leg base of support, progressing the difficulty of the core stability and muscle recruitment in the hamstrings and glutes.

A keen understanding of the rules will help you refine your workout to the precise difficulty level each time—not too easy, not resulting in mechanical breakdown, but challenging enough to produce the best results. Your goal is to be better in each successive workout.

Stability Ball Progressions

There are numerous methods of progressing the level of difficulty when using stability ball exercises. Specific structured progressions are included in the text of each exercise. But knowing several guidelines for simplifying or advancing an exercise will allow you to modify each exercise many times over to define the most appropriate level of challenge for you. If you are uncertain, you should choose regressions to ensure that you complete the exercise safely within your current abilities. However, when you are experienced with an exercise and begin to find it easy, adopt progressions to make sure you are challenged. If an exercise is not challenging, you will not stimulate improvement. With this in mind, the following are points that you can consider when regressing or progressing your exercises.

Change the base of support. By decreasing the base of support for an exercise, you can increase the challenge of balance, which makes leg, glute, and torso musculature work much harder. You can accomplish this by increasing the inflation of the ball, which will result in a smaller base of ball support. You can also change the base of support by moving from a four-point support to a three- or two-point support. An example of a four-point support is a stability ball push-up in which you have both hands on the ball and both feet on the floor. To increase the level of difficulty in the push-up, you can use a three-point base of support by raising one foot off the floor. You can also decrease your base of support by placing your hands and feet closer together. Although you are still in a four-point base of support, this move results in a decreased overall base of support.

Change the length of the lever. As you alter the length of your lever arm from short to long, you increase the difficulty of the exercise, as with the abdominal crunch medicine ball throw. Throwing from the chest is easier than using a longer lever and throwing from overhead. Your trunk can also be the lever arm between the floor and where you make contact with the ball. Rollouts (chapter 4) connect the toes or knees on the floor, with the hands on the ball, by stiffening the torso and arms. A short rollout is easier than a longer rollout. Supine bridges (chapter 4) place feet on the floor as a base of support and upper back atop the ball. Legs, glutes, and torso keep the hips up and connect the feet and upper back. A short ball bridge is easier than a longer one. Minor changes in these body positions can make a dramatic difference in level of difficulty by changing the coordination, effort, or force required. Notice even changing an inch or two dramatically increases the muscle tension. Good mechanics and minor changes to body position can magnify the muscle response and amplify your results.

Increase range of motion.   By increasing movements from a smaller to a larger range of motion, you can increase the difficulty of the exercise, as with the push-up with hands on ball. You can progress from partial push-ups to full-range push-ups.

Change the speed of movement.   Changing the tempo of an exercise changes the result. Very slow movements keep the muscle loaded under tension longer and help build strength and stability. Fast dynamic movements tend to build power. The tempo of movement also makes the exercise easier or more difficult. Most experts suggest that moving faster is more difficult. But there is no general rule here. Some exercises done more quickly are much more difficult. Still other exercises done very slowly require much more strength and balance. Know that speed of movement alters the demands. You will need to adjust your tempo on an exercise to learn whether it results in an easier or more difficult execution. The surprise may be that slower is harder.

Add resistance.   You can increase the intensity of an exercise by adding some form of loaded resistance, such as a medicine ball, an external free-weight, cable, or elastic tubing, as with the jackknife exercise with a cable attached to the legs (chapter 4). Strength tubing needs to be long enough to accommodate whole-body moves in strength ball training. It also needs to be strong enough to offer enough resistance. It should come with a protective sleeve to make the tubing more durable and, if it does eventually break, to ensure it coils inside the sleeve instead of snapping back and hitting you.

Close the eyes.   By closing your eyes, you increase the proprioceptive demand in the body, flooding other sensors and receptors positioned to give feedback on changes to muscles, ligaments, tendons, and joint position. Removing visual feedback overloads your proprioceptive system, forcing those "minibrains" to work harder and improve. This adds a level of difficulty, but you should take caution. Some exercises, such as kneeling on the ball, will require spotting by a strength coach.

Medicine Ball Progressions

Selecting the correct medicine ball load and modifying the method of applying the medicine ball contribute to making an exercise level appropriate.

Increase ball weight.   As strength and power improve, selecting a heavier medicine ball will progress the amount of overload placed on the muscles, stimulating further adaptations.

Introduce throwing variables.   With a ball of the same weight, increase the distance between partners. This requires more power on the throw and more coordination and eccentric strength on the catch. Or move closer together and increase the catch–throw speed. This requires reactions and eye–hand coordination and shifts the emphasis to power, training the eccentric–concentric coupling.

Use a single arm.   Changing from two-hand catches to single-hand catches increases the reliance on the core, hips, and legs, along with the posterior chain, to absorb the load. In general, it increases the complexity of the exercise, forcing greater whole-body involvement.

Use vision tracking.   For exercises with a medicine ball, locking vision on the ball as it travels increases the balance challenge. For example, stand on one leg while passing the ball overhead, or move it from one side of the body to the other. Think of tunnel vision, seeing nothing but the ball. If you also add a head tilt—tilting your head back to look up at the ball overhead—the level of balance difficulty is heightened.

Integrate movement or balance.   Adding movement to whole-body exercises or instability will increase the metabolic cost, coordination required, muscle activation, number of muscles recruited, and transferability.

Make the exercise unpredictable.   Throwing the ball at varied times or throwing the ball to different positions requires quick reactions, quick thinking, and quick body adjustments to nail the mechanics needed for a whole-body catch. For example, in partner passes, pass the ball to the right, left, up high, down low, and overhead. Mixing it up is fun and makes the muscles more responsive.

Selecting Training Tools

Stability balls can now be found in just about any type of store—department stores, supermarkets, and even drugstores. With so many choices of balls, how can you determine which one might be appropriate for you? The following tells you everything you need to know.

Sizing of Stability Balls

Most manufacturers of stability balls make sizing recommendations based on your height. One general rule is that when you sit on the ball, your thighs should be parallel to the floor. If they are below the parallel level, you will be forced to use poor posture for many of the exercises. In many cases, this rule is a good general guideline to use when determining your ball size. But as you will see in the exercise descriptions, this rule does not always hold true. Many exercises use a variety of ball sizes through their progressions. In your training facility you should have several various-sized balls available.

For personal use, those who are 5 feet 10 inches to 6 feet 3 inches (178 to 190 cm) tall can accomplish most exercises with 55-centimeter and 65-centimeter balls. Those who are 5 feet 9 inches or shorter (175 cm or less) can use 45-centimeter and 55-centimeter balls. Those who are 6 feet 4 inches or taller (193 cm or taller) can work with 65-centimeter and 75-centimeter balls.

Quality of Stability Balls

Stability balls have become a more common training tool in the mainstream populations, and mass merchandisers now stock the product on a regular basis. With many more options than in the past, shoppers are able to choose from bargain-basement balls at general retailers to specialty balls off the Internet. You should shop for quality. This is a tool that must support your body weight and handle the rigors of physical training. If the ball looks and feels on the thin side, like a beach ball, you can assume it is a cheaper product. If it feels thicker, it might be of good quality.

The accurate measure is in the ABS rating. Stability balls are labeled ABS if they are truly an "antiburst" ball. When a ball is punctured, ABS balls will slowly deflate instead of bursting immediately, even when you're sitting atop the ball with your body mass and holding weights. Balls that are lab tested are assigned a weight they can handle and still demonstrate reliable antiburst properties. Look for a ball with an ABS rating for 300 pounds (136 kg) or more. Balls are also tested for the total amount of weight they can support. This is usually about three times their ABS rating. A 300-pound ABS ball could hold 900 pounds (408 kg). For more information on stability balls, search at www.twistconditioning.com for quality assurance.

BOSU Dynamic Stabilizing Load (DSL) Balls

BOSU is an acronym for both sides up. DSL stands for dynamic stabilizing load. One example is the Ballast ball, which was invented by David Weck, creator of the BOSU Balance Trainer. Weck's training tools allow coaches and exercise practitioners to create new exercises. The dynamic stabilizing load inside the ball is a granular substance that provides stability when the ball sits on the floor, a load to lift when the ball is carried off the floor, and a perturbation when the DSL shifts from side to side.

Options in Medicine Balls

Similar to dumbbells, medicine balls come in various weights. Most women and kids will handle a 4-, 6-, or 8-pound ball (about 2, 3, and 4 kg, respectively). Men most often select an 8- or 10-pound ball (about 4 or 5 kg). For some exercises, elite athletes use 25- and 30-pound balls (about 12 and 14 kg, respectively). (Note that these metric conversions for ball weights are not precise. That is, a 2-kilogram ball is actually 4.4 pounds. Some brands of medicine balls are available in metric weights only, and some are available in English weights only.) Try some exercises in the gym or with your personal trainer to get a better idea of the weight range best suited to your strength level. Having at least two medicine balls, one of medium and one of heavy weight, will accommodate many exercises. Once you have a set weight to work with, there are several ways to make a drill more difficult, even with a ball of the same weight.

Several kinds of medicine balls are available. They all produce the dynamic load required for building strength, so make your choice based on individual preference for their other features. Original medicine balls were big and leather bound. You can also select rubber medicine balls that are slightly smaller than a basketball. PowerBounce medicine balls are constructed of thick rubber and are virtually indestructible, and they bounce off the floor or wall. Today many people opt for soft-shell fitness balls. They are small and soft, so they can be gripped in one hand. They're also great for tracking exercises. Some people find them softer to catch. For more information on medicine balls, go to www.twistconditioning.com for quality assurance and author recommendations, or check out a specialty fitness retailer.

Technique Notes

As strength and conditioning coaches, we have more than 40 combined years of experience in working with professional athletes and more than 60 combined years of experience in fitness. Enforcing proper technique has been the foundation of our success. Do not settle for anything less when you are training yourself or your clients. A component that is common to every exercise in *Strength Ball Training* is the concept of setting the core. You will achieve greater levels of stability and strength if you can master this technique and use it as you train yourself or coach your clients.

Setting the Abdominals

Since the first edition of *Strength Ball Training* there has been much debate about the optimal method of setting the core to provide a solid pillar for completing exercise movements. Setting the abdominals is a simple yet important technique in the setup phase of all stability ball and medicine ball exercises. Slightly drawing in your navel toward your spine and giving your pelvis an anterior tilt (which emphasizes the natural curve in your lower back) accomplishes the setting of the abdominals. This drawing in serves a significant function. Most important, it initiates a support mechanism for the spine and torso as a result of the transverse abdominis and internal oblique muscles being activated. This motion of drawing in has been demonstrated to assist in the reduction of compression on the spine by as much as 40 percent as well as promoting the natural function of these muscles. When this contraction is activated, it provides your body with a much more stable core area for executing all exercises (Richardson et al. 1999; Wirhed 1990).

In the third edition of Stuart McGill's book *Low Back Disorders* (2015), he emphasizes a technique known as bracing, which is an isometric contraction that results in coactivation of the obliques and transverse abdominis. McGill states that this method provides increased stability, and it more readily prepares the body for unexpected loads. He also claims that it provides for a greater base of pull for muscles than the hollowing, or drawing-in, technique, which decreases the base. It has been our experience that a combination of the two techniques brings about a more solid core. This would involve a slight hollowing of the abdominals along with a slight isometric contraction.

We cue our athletes to contract 360 degrees around the core to set the core. With younger kids, to help them achieve the sensation of bracing, we have fun faking a punch to the belly—at which they instinctively brace. It is a simple way to establish the isometric contraction. For older clients, we make the analogy of a corset so that they sense a stabilized trunk before each exercise. Whatever the cue, a blend of drawing in and bracing sets the core to absorb and produce loadings and to provide a better base from which the arms and legs can generate force. With training, this will become natural. After weeks of strength ball training, you will notice that you begin to automatically set the core for tasks outside the gym, such as reaching to lift a heavy object off a shelf or skiing on very difficult mogul runs. Enjoy your results applied during day-to-day tasks and in your favorite sport!

Precautions

One of the issues that we have seen since the release of the first edition of *Strength Ball Training* is a misuse of some exercise progressions. As good as the ball looks for increasing core strength and stability, there are instances in which it should not be used. Two of these instances are in people with chronic low back pain and those who are just beginning a strengthening program. These recommendations are grounded in the fact that increased activation of the core musculature also involves an increase in spinal loads. That is not necessarily a bad thing, but proper progression will ultimately ensure against any kind of injury. It has been suggested that the proper progression would involve the use of stable surfaces and then progress to unstable surfaces (McGill 1998). Introduce unstable surfaces such as stability balls only once you or your client has sufficient spinal stability to be able to accept loads that will challenge the core without pain during and after the exercise. You may want to spend 3 to 8 weeks doing exercises on stable surfaces before progressing to the greater challenge of stability ball training.

The following are a few stable exercises that we recommend if you are beginning a program. You should be able to do these exercises comfortably before progressing to the more advanced unstable exercises.

Figure 2.1 demonstrates the static back extension. Hold the body in perfect alignment so that there is a line from the ear to the shoulder, hips, and knee. There should be a very slight bend in the knees during this exercise. Do not allow the knees to hyperextend, which can place undue stress on the backs of the knees. Your goal for this exercise is to hold the position for 2 to

3 minutes. Do not start your program by attempting to complete long sets. Begin with sets of 30 seconds and slowly progress weekly by adding 10 to 15 seconds to each set.

Figure 2.2 shows the McGill static side raise, also known as the static side plank. McGill has done much research on spinal biomechanics. (See the third edition of his book *Low Back Disorders*, 2015, for more information.) Again, as you can see in the setup, there should be a fairly straight line from the head all the way to the feet. You may find it too difficult to begin this move from the feet. If so, try flexing the knees to 90 degrees and eventually progress to straight legs. Your goal for this is to hold the position for 90 to 120 seconds. Begin with sets of 30 seconds and slowly progress weekly by adding 10 to 15 seconds to each set.

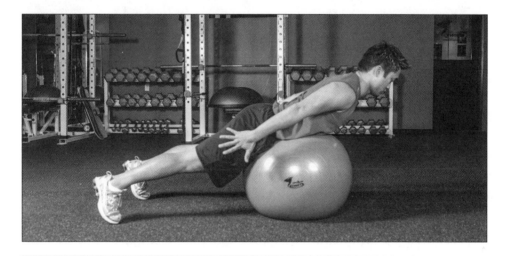

Figure 2.1 Static back extension.

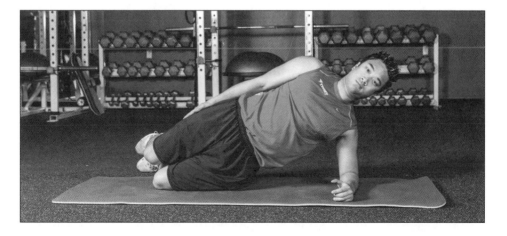

Figure 2.2 McGill static side raise.

Figure 2.3 shows the single-leg hip lift. While lying on your back, flex at one hip and hold this position with your arms. The opposite knee should be flexed so that your foot is flat on the floor. Set your core and press your foot into the floor to raise your hips off the floor. Press up to a point where you have a line from your knee to the hip to the shoulder. Your goal for this movement is to be able to complete at least 10 repetitions on each side with good form.

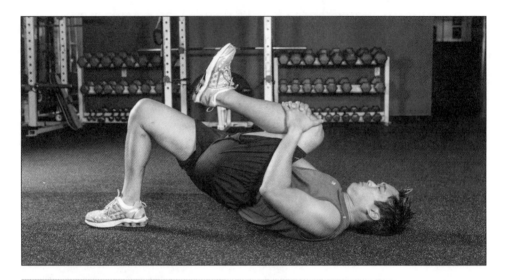

Figure 2.3   Single-leg hip lift.

If you want to train your core while focusing on other body parts, you should consider exercises that focus on using single-arm movements. For athletes preparing for high-force dynamic movement and for fitness enthusiasts who strength train, the intersegmental and stabilizing muscles must be well developed to prevent injury. These intersegmental and stabilizing muscles in the spine, shoulders, hips, knees, and ankles can best be stimulated and overloaded by performing exercises in an unstable environment. The stability ball provides this very environment, which will give you several viable options to enhance your exercise toolkit.

Common Terms

As you use the exercises in this book, you will encounter some common terms that describe positions or movements:

Tabletop, or **bridge**, is the act of lying on the ball with your head and shoulders supported, feet under your knees, and core engaged. In this position you will resemble a tabletop or bridge.

Supine involves lying on the back or with your face upward. When you lie on your bed on your back you are in a supine position.

Prone involves lying on your front or facing the floor. When you lie on your bed on your belly, you are in a prone position.

Static means no movement. So an exercise requiring a static hold would result in the contraction of muscles with no movement produced.

Throughout the book you will see numbers designating **tempo**, such as 1:1:1 tempo. Each digit represents a phase of the movement. In this example are three phases, and each phase is to be held for one second. Generally the first number represents the lowering, or the eccentric portion, of the lift. The middle number represents the middle position of the range of motion, and the final number is the speed of the concentric portion, or the raising of the weight.

The concepts that we have covered in this chapter may seem elementary, but they are critical to your success in executing the exercises described in the book. These foundational concepts will lead you down the path of success with your programming.

CHAPTER 3

ASSESSMENT

The fitness test can be intimidating for many people who are just beginning to participate in a fitness program. Some would even describe it as a barrier to engaging in fitness. The fear of the dreaded test—pushing yourself to the max, finding out how "fat" you are or weak you might be—is not an appealing experience for most people, let alone someone who is intimidated by the whole milieu of fitness. This is one of the reasons we avoid using the term *test* and instead use the more user-friendly term *fitness assessment*.

Having been involved in the NHL as strength and conditioning coaches for many years, we have evaluated the results of many NHL testing sessions. We have also evaluated thousands of nonathletes seeking to be fit and healthy. The problem lies in what aspects to evaluate in order to benefit the client. Some professionals in the industry believe the more assessments, the better. We believe that evaluation for sport performance and fitness is an act that is observed every day with every movement a client performs—from the moment he or she steps in the door, to the beginning of the warm-up, to the end of the very last set. If you are a trainer, this is important because there are many points of movement to observe that might dictate a small change in the program. For example, your client may have played a tough soccer game the night before and as she walks into the gym, you might notice that one shoulder is more elevated. With one of our pro athletes we might manually treat the issue, determine if there are some exercises we can use to help relieve the tightness causing this, or augment the program to reduce stress in that area. The bottom line is that if you allow a client to train with an issue that might impede proper movement of a joint, then you are teaching that person to reinforce that same improper movement or posture. As Stuart McGill notes in the third edition of his book *Low Back Disorders* (2015), "Tissue overload causes damage and subsequent low back troubles" (p. 167). This can certainly be applied to many other areas of the body. It is beyond the scope of this book to delve deeply into this area, but it surely is something you should be concerned about if you are a trainer. If you are using this book as a tool for engaging in a new program, be aware of how you feel and how you look in the mirror, and realize that pain or the inability to complete a movement that you once did with ease is a sign to back off and check in with a professional.

Sometimes a poor score does not indicate you are weak in the specific muscles you are testing. The cause may be a supporting muscle group that is not doing its intended job. An example is the movement of a simple push-up. Some of the muscles that are key to an effective push-up are those that you cannot even see. For example, the subscapularis and serratus anterior are muscles that assist in stabilizing the shoulder blade against the posterior rib cage. When these muscles are not functioning, the shoulder blade may wing off the rib cage and not support the movement of the push-up very effectively. The result might be pain in the shoulder or an inability to reach full range of motion in the shoulder. So if you or your client has a poor result in a push-up test, it does not necessarily mean that you have weak pectorals or triceps. There could be a fault that you may not specifically see during such a test. Issues like this can be observed only via manual muscle testing. It is beyond the scope of this chapter to delve into this further, but an excellent resource on the topic is Ken Kinakin's book *Optimal Muscle Training* (2008).

The assessment tools provide you with some baseline data that will assist you in understanding where you rate and the areas you should focus on. The data will provide you with a good indicator of your core health, among other things. A strong and stable core will provide you with the foundation for executing efficient and precise movements in your strength ball training program.

Total-Body Strength and Stability Assessment

This assessment looks at how the whole body functions through a combination of a strength movement in the upper body and no movement in the rest of the body—that is, the lower body must remain still in a strong and stable position.

Setup

Begin by starting in a push-up position, feet hip-width apart and hands just slightly outside shoulder width. Women set up from the knees. A partner or instructor places a dowel along the participant's back, making contact with the glutes, thoracic spine (upper back), and head. This position must be held at all times during the execution of the test (see figure *a*).

Movement

Starting at the top of the push-up position, the partner turns on a metronome at 50 beats per minute. This pace will result in half the push-up movement being completed every 1.66 seconds, or up and down in 3.32 seconds. If you do not have a metronome, there are many available at no cost online. With each tick of the metronome, you should be at either end of the movement. The goal for the bottom position is to lower to 2.5 inches (6.35 cm) off the floor (a tennis ball could be used as a guide).

During the movement, the partner should ensure that the participant is keeping all three points of contact with the dowel (see figure *b*) and will count the number of push-ups completed.

Finish

Completion of the test will be determined when one of the following occurs:

1. One of the points of contact with the dowel changes (such as arch increases in the lower back, head drops).
2. Participant cannot keep pace with beats.

Average Score

Men: 20

Women: 21

We conducted this whole-body strength and stability assessment on a nonathletic but physically active population. The ages ranged from 20 to 47, and the above data were designated as standards of this population. (Note that competitive athletes may obtain higher scores.)

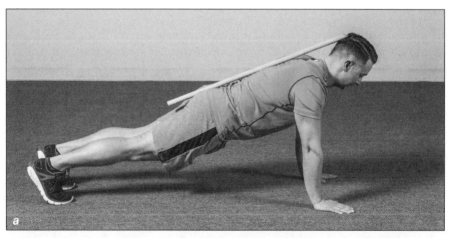

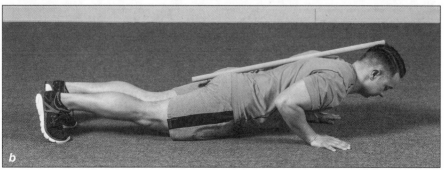

Core Endurance and Mobility Assessments

The core endurance assessments are simple yet effective methods of looking at core strength and stability. Unlike the total-body strength and stability assessment that assesses upper-body strength with the core, these three focus on the core in the frontal and sagittal planes. Stuart McGill's third edition of *Low Back Disorders* (2015) refers to these assessments as having showed very high reliability when repeated over multiple days. This is important when identifying weaknesses that can be addressed with specific exercises. McGill also indicates that those at risk for low back pain are people with poor muscular endurance of the torso flexors, lateral musculature, and back extensors.

   McGill's work over the years has been proven to be exceptional. Along with what we have seen from a practical standpoint with our general clients and athletes, we are confident that these core endurance assessments will add great value to your pursuit of strength and health.

Lateral Core Musculature Assessment

This assessment (known as side plank or isometric lateral bridge) assesses the core muscles of the frontal plane. Note that the key here is the goal of having both sides equal.

Setup

Get into a full side plank with the top arm across the chest and top foot in front of the bottom foot in a toe-to-heel alignment. Support is provided by the elbow and feet.

Movement

Brace the abdominals and lift the hips off the floor to create a straight line from the shoulders to the hips and all the way to the feet. Count the number of seconds the position is held.

Finish

The assessment ends at the first sign of the hips dropping or any kind of rotation of the body. Repeat on the other side.

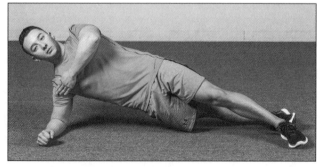

Average Score

   Men: 95-100 seconds

   Women: 83-86 seconds

Back Extension Assessment

This assessment can be performed on a massage table with straps or on a back extension bench. This test has been called the Biering-Sorenson test, named after the first research on the related to back pain.

Setup

The hips, pelvis, and ankles should be secured as shown. The placement of the hips should be so that the anterior superior iliac spine of the pelvis is supported at the edge of the bench. Hands are crossed under the chest and head is in neutral position.

Movement

There is no movement. Count the number of seconds the position is held.

Finish

The assessment is terminated if there is pain or any kind of drop from the initial setup position or if 240 seconds have passed.

Average Score

Men: 160 seconds

Women: 173 seconds

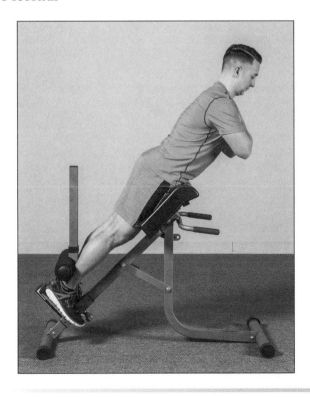

Flexor Endurance Assessment

This assessment looks at the anterior side of the core, mainly the abdominals, in a static sit-up posture.

Setup

The back should be set at an angle of 60 degrees (use a goniometer to determine) and the feet should be secured. Both the knees and hips should be locked in at 90-degree angles.

Movement

This position should be held with no movement. Count the number of seconds the position is held.

Finish

Any backward movement of more than 4 inches (10 cm) indicates the test is over.

Average Score

Men: 136 seconds

Women: 134 seconds

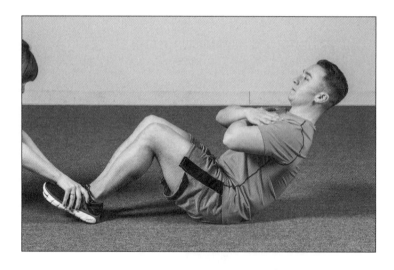

Overhead Squat Assessment

The overhead squat is part of functional movement screening (FMS) made popular by Grey Cook. Although we are not using the full screening parameters of the FMS, we like this movement as an assessment and an exercise because it requires effort from every major joint in the body. It is a full-body movement with great emphasis on the legs, hips, lower and upper back, and shoulders. It allows you or your trainer to determine if you have any movement problems bilaterally (both sides), or unilaterally (if you favor one side) and detect which joint may be the limiting factor. Because strength ball training is so integrated and functional, the overhead squat is a go-to movement for us. If you do not have a coach or trainer to work with, here is how to assess yourself and the key points you should be aware of.

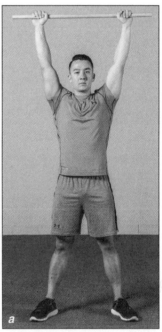

Setup

Place feet slightly wider than shoulder-width apart with your hands holding a dowel so that, when your elbows are bent, they are at a 90-degree angle. Once you have this set, push the dowel overhead into an extended arm and shoulder position (see figure *a*).

Movement

From this standing position, lower yourself slowly into a squat where your thighs are just below horizontal (see figure *b*). Maintain contact with your heels on the floor, knees over your feet, head facing forward, and chest up, all the while keeping the dowel fully extended overhead and centered between your heels and toes. Give yourself three or four chances to get it right.

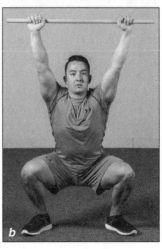

If your squat is done with your chest up, your thighs parallel to the floor, and your feet on the ground, score yourself a 3. If you cannot achieve the technique, place a small riser or plank under your heels and repeat. Score a 2 if your knees are still not aligned as indicated or the dowel is past your feet. Score a 1 if there is too much forward lean, the upper thigh is not below horizontal, the knees are past the toes, or lumbar flexion (arching of the back) is seen. If there is any pain, score a 0 and have a professional assess you. Pain may be an indicator of a deeper problem limiting this movement.

Corrective Action for Malalignment in Overhead Squat

Ankle Dorsiflexion

Try these stretches, flexing the ankles in a slow pumping action, or hold for 15 to 20 seconds. You can do the stretches either standing (see figure *a*) or sitting (see figure *b*).

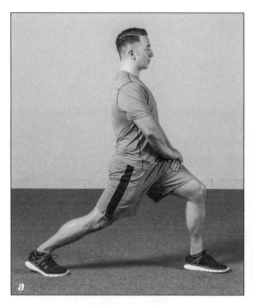
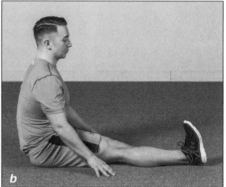

Deep Squat Progression

Try the deep squat progression (see figures *a-c*). Standing on an incline, squat deep, touching your left hand to the floor and raising your right hand to the ceiling. Repeat on the opposite side. Or try the wall slide (see figures *d-f*) in a controlled manner if you have restrictions in the shoulder or thoracic spine. Standing against a wall, raise your arms straight overhead. Move your arms slowly down the wall so that forearms are parallel to the floor and then at a 45-degree angle.

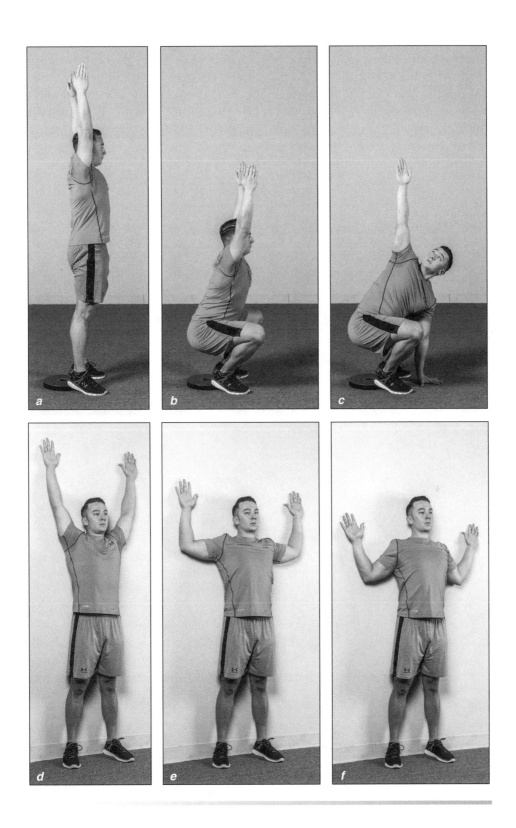

The assessments in this chapter provide some simple guidelines as you prepare yourself or your clients for exercises in the book. It is beyond the scope of this chapter to completely detail exercise progressions from a correction standpoint. You can use the assessments as a gauge for improvement and a motivational tool for reaching new goals. Attainable goals are those that will continue to foster engagement and improvement in fitness. In the event that you or a client is not comfortable or in unreasonable pain while performing the assessments, you should stop and consult with a health professional.

CHAPTER 4

CORE STABILIZATION

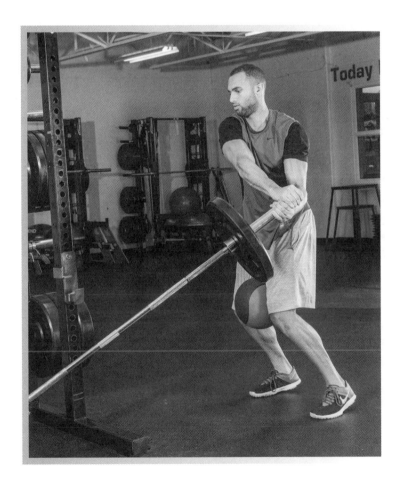

Jackknife

To shift the load to your lower abdominals and hip flexors, add this exercise to your program. It requires upper-body and core stability and activates the lower abs and hip muscles to draw the ball in toward the body. The weight in your lower body is transferred through the ball to produce a load against the hip flexors.

Setup

Standing behind the ball, crouch down and place your abdomen on top of the ball. Roll forward until your hands reach the floor in front of the ball. Walk your hands out until only your feet remain on top of the ball. Contract the core to hold a strong link. Your body should be in a straight and firm line from feet to head.

Movement

From the prone push-up position, keep the legs straight and bend at the waist so the hips elevate and the knees move closer to the torso. This moves the ball toward your hands. Keep the speed of movement under control, with a 1:1:1 tempo.

Finish

Extend your legs to move the ball back to the start position. At this point, at the end of each rep, your body should be linked with strong contractions forming one level, straight line.

Tips and Progressions

- One method of progression is to add resistance to the ankles. You can accomplish this by adding a cable or strength tubing. So as you flex your hips forward, you are pulling on not only the ball but also the resistance of the cable.

- Another progression is a modified one-leg bent-knee jackknife. In this version, begin with only one foot on the ball. The right leg is off the ball yet straight and firm. Draw the ball up toward your chest with your lower abdominals and hip flexors. Balance on one leg in this position, holding your contraction, before straightening the left leg back to the setup position, following a 1:2:1 tempo.

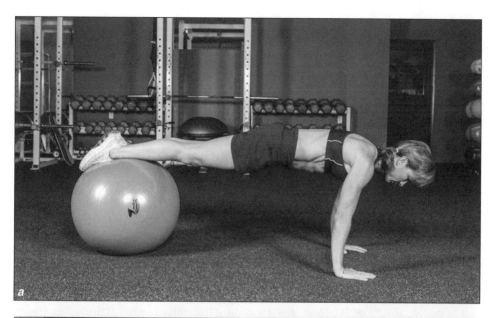

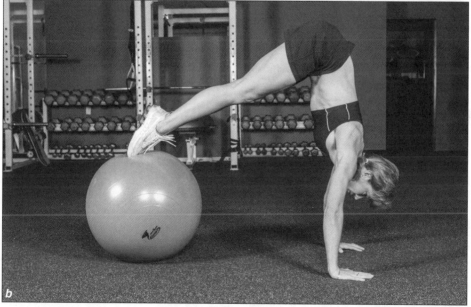

Prone Balance

The prone balance is also known by some as a prone plank position. It provides a challenge to the core in the sagittal plane.

Setup

Roll out on a stability ball so that it is set under your elbows in a prone position. You should be propped up on your elbows, with your shoulders placed directly over your elbows. Engage your core to create a slight kyphotic posture (back rounded) and hold this position. Your feet should be hip-width apart.

Movement and Finish

There is no real movement for the prone balance because it is a static exercise. Hold the described position for 30 to 120 seconds.

Tips and Progressions

- You can use many progressions during this exercise. The first to consider is foot placement. Progress from a hip-width stance to a narrow stance or single-leg stance.
- Change the effective lever arm by rolling the ball forward, from side to side, in circles, and in figure eights.
- Add resistance by wearing a weight vest or placing a sandbag over the low back.
- You can achieve greater instability by placing the feet on top of a BOSU or balance board.
- Also see prone ball hold with knee drive (chapter 6) as a variation with some hip movement.

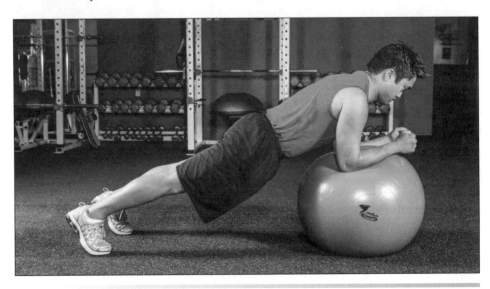

McGill Side Raise
With Static Hip Adduction

This exercise is named after Stuart McGill, one of the world's leading spine researchers, from the University of Waterloo. This movement focuses on core musculature in the frontal plane while incorporating the hip adductors.

Setup

Lie sideways on a mat with your elbow propping up your body. You should have your body set so you are supported laterally. Place a stability ball between your feet and squeeze to fire your adductors on your hips.

Movement

Engage your core and laterally lift your body off the floor, maintaining the adductor contraction on the ball. There should be a fairly straight line from your ear to shoulder, hips, and knees. Hold the contracted position one to two seconds.

Finish

After holding the contracted position, lower yourself back to the starting position. As you lower your hips back down, do not allow your body to rest. At about a centimeter from the floor, begin your next lift. Repeat on the opposite side after reps are completed.

Tips and Progressions

- To work static strength and stability of your core, try static holds in the contracted position. Holds can be anywhere from 30 to 90 seconds in length on each side.
- Add extra resistance by placing a sandbag or weight vest over your hips.

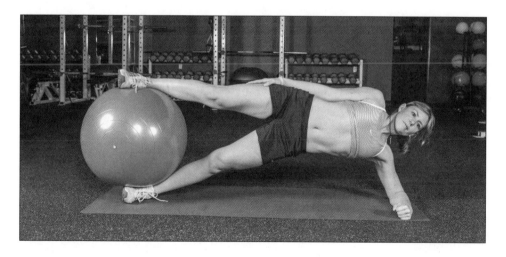

Prone Balance Hip Opener

The prone balance hip opener is similar to the prone balance. It adds the component of hip mobility to the prone balance and changes the balance challenge of the push-up position hip opener from the feet to the arms.

Setup

Roll out on a stability ball so that you are in a prone position with the ball set under your elbows. You should be propped up on your elbows with your shoulders directly over your elbows.

Movement

Flex one hip forward to create a 90-degree angle. Adduct the leg as far as you can, squeeze this position for a second, then abduct out to the side.

Finish

Complete a set number of reps and then switch legs.

Tips and Progressions

- Increase the challenge of this movement by adding a hip extension after each hip rotation. To do this, after you have abducted the hip and returned to the start position, extend the hip straight back, hold, return to the start position, then proceed with hip adduction.
- Add resistance by putting weights on your ankle.

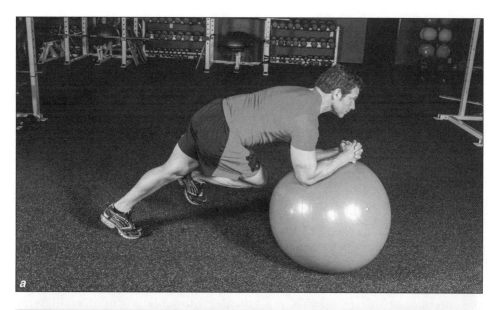

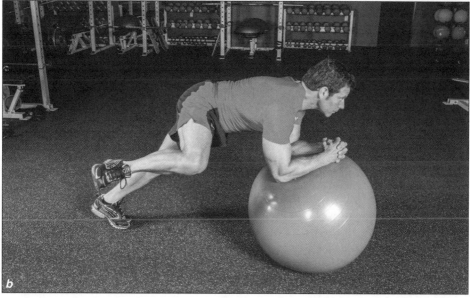

Bridge T Fall-Off

The bridge is a key position that dozens of exercises build from. Bridge fall-offs activate the deep abdominal muscles and all core muscles to hold the bridge, brake before falling, and pull back into position. It works 360 degrees around the torso.

Setup

Sit on top of the ball and slowly roll forward so your hips move off the ball. Continue until your middle back is on top of the ball. You will feel your shoulder blades at the top or middle of the ball. Your feet are flat on the floor and shoulder-width apart, upper legs parallel to the floor. The key to a functional bridge is to elevate your hips to form a straight line from neck to knees. Be sure to hold your hips up strong. Raise your arms out to the side so that your torso and arms make a T position.

Movement

Slowly shift your weight to one side, rolling out onto your triceps. Keep your hips up, not allowing any rotation at the hips or shoulders. Move as far to the side as you can without losing your solid position and without falling off the ball.

Finish

Using your core muscles, pull your body back across the ball until your shoulder blades are back on top of the ball. Continue to move through to the opposite side and repeat the movement.

Tips and Progressions

- Place a dowel across the chest from shoulder to shoulder to evaluate stability and body alignment. Any hip or torso rotation will be evident when the dowel rolls or tips and falls off.

- Successful execution of bridge fall-offs can lead to reaction fall-offs. When your partner lightly pushes you to the left or the right, you must react and decelerate the movement with your core muscles, reversing the movement before falling off the ball. This is more sportlike because you are not worried as much about strict technique as you are about producing the resulting function. You will tend to roll your torso when pushed to the extreme side ranges before braking and returning to your middle setup position.

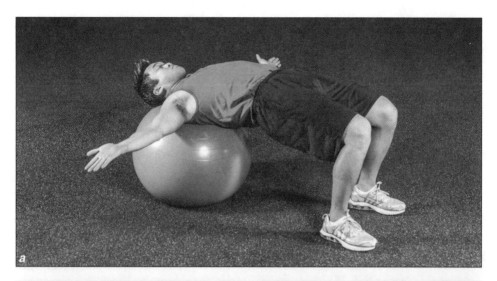

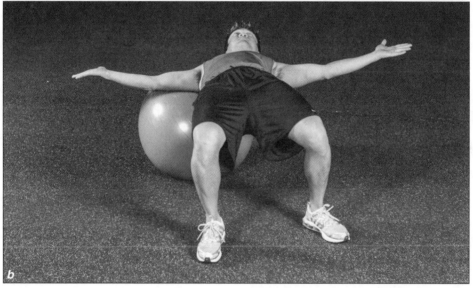

Supine Stabilizer Scissors

Although it has a similar name as supine rotator scissors in chapter 5, the main difference here is that supine stabilizer scissors uses the ball as a base of support and focuses on strength in the sagittal plane.

Setup

Place a ball in front of something solid that you can grip on to—either a power rack or a solid piece of equipment. The height you have to grasp is approximately hip height. Lie back over the stability ball so it provides support to your low back. Reach back and grasp the bar with extended arms. Your legs should also be extended and parallel with the floor.

Movement

Begin movement by raising one leg straight up and lowering the opposite leg approximately 10 to 15 degrees.

Finish

Hold this position for a second and then reverse your legs.

Tips and Progressions

This movement provides a great challenge to the low back and abdominals from a stability standpoint. If you feel pain during this movement, it might be a result of your not having the required base strength to maintain your position. In this case, you can try the movement with bent knees.

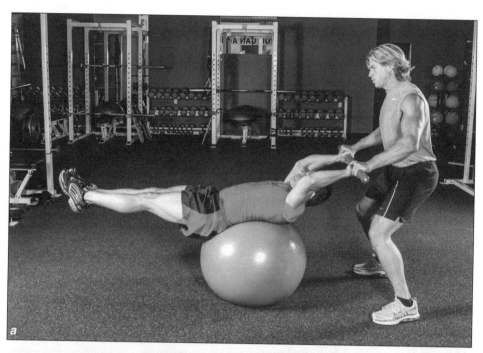

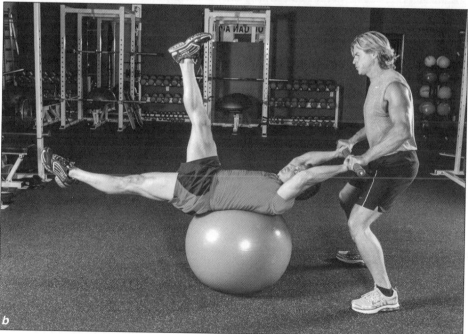

Bridge With Medicine Ball Drops

This exercise requires the core muscles to eccentrically decelerate the falling load (medicine ball) while producing stabilization to hold the basic bridge and to balance and return to balance after catching the ball.

Setup

Sit on top of the ball and slowly roll forward so your hips move off the ball. Continue until your middle back is on top of the ball. Your shoulder blades will be at the top or middle of the ball. Your feet are flat on the floor and shoulder-width apart, and upper legs are parallel to the floor. The key to a functional bridge is to elevate your hips to form a straight line from neck to knees. Hold your hips up strong. Extend your arms up above your chest, with your hands ready in a catching position.

Movement

Your partner stands in front of you, lightly tossing a medicine ball so it drops outside of your center of gravity. You must rotate slightly and catch the ball as it drops to the right or left of your chest area. Catch the ball while keeping your hips up.

Finish

Brake, balance, and throw the ball back to your partner before using your core to return to the setup position in preparation for the next rep.

Tips and Progressions

- Randomize the medicine ball tosses from left to right, above shoulder to waist level, as well as overhead.
- Give the spotter feedback if you can handle more challenging drops.
- Likewise, the spotter needs to remind you to keep your hips up strong and bring the feet back to the starting stance. Most people automatically widen their stance when catching the ball instead of relying on their core strength.
- To increase the difficulty of the exercise, bring your feet together.

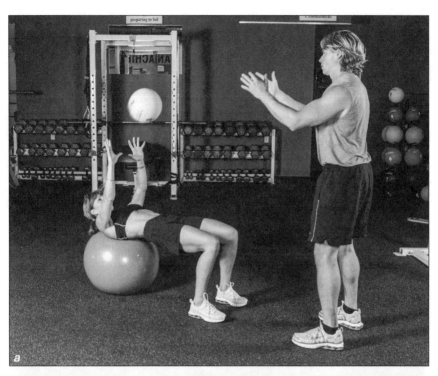

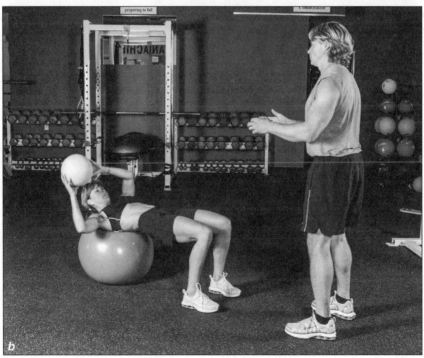

Bridge Ball Hug

The bridge ball hug introduces the concept of static and dynamic contractions in the same exercise.

Setup

Sit on top of the ball and slowly roll forward so your hips move off the ball. Continue until your middle back is on top of the ball. Your shoulder blades will be at the top middle of the ball. Your feet are flat on the floor and shoulder-width apart, and upper legs are parallel to the floor. The key to a functional bridge is to elevate your hips to form a straight line from neck to knees. Hold your hips up strong. Place another ball on your chest, wrapping your arms around the ball as if you were hugging the ball.

Movement

Maintain your setup position while a partner begins slapping the ball in multiple angles. The key is to hug the ball as tightly as possible and limit movement of your body and ball during the slaps. Setting your abdominals during this exercise will assist in stabilizing your body.

Finish

This exercise is finished when you complete the total number of slaps in a set; 20 to 30 slaps are recommended.

Tips and Progressions

Increase the difficulty by holding the ball away from your body with arms extended over your chest.

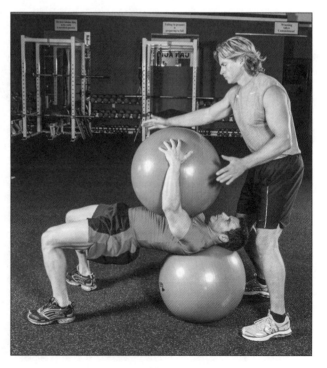

Kneeling Ball Self-Pass and Tracking

This is a fun exercise that forces participants to think their way through with keen body awareness.

Setup

Begin kneeling up on the ball—glutes up off the heels, torso up tall, back in a neutral position with the core muscles engaged.

Movement

Start by passing the medicine ball back and forth from one hand to the other with arms out in front of you. Progress by taking the passes up overhead.

Tips and Progressions

- Start off with small short passes and progress to wider passes.
- Progress further by tunneling vision to just the ball as it travels from side to side in front of the body and also up overhead and across to the other side.

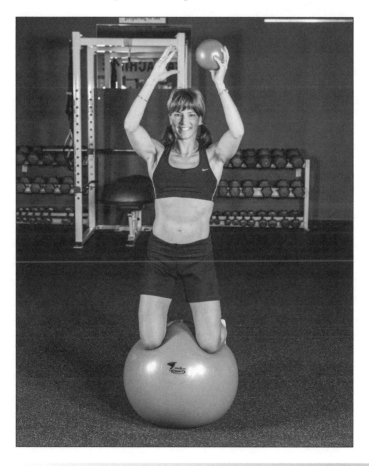

Standing Bar Twist
With Medicine Ball Squeeze

This is a challenging movement that combines core stabilization with your arms acting as loading levers. The tie-in for the lower body comes in the static medicine ball squeeze that works the adductors along with the core musculature to enhance the link between obliques and adductors.

Setup

With a loaded bar wedged in the base of a wall or squat rack, pick up the bar; in a hand-over-hand position, the bar should be at about mouth level. Have a partner set the medicine ball between your legs for the squeeze.

Movement

Maintain a stable core as you let your arms slowly drop to one side while squeezing the legs.

Finish

Return all the way to the other side without stopping at the midposition.

Tips and Progressions

- The bar should be in a continuous slow and controlled motion for the complete set.
- Add plates to the bar to increase the load.

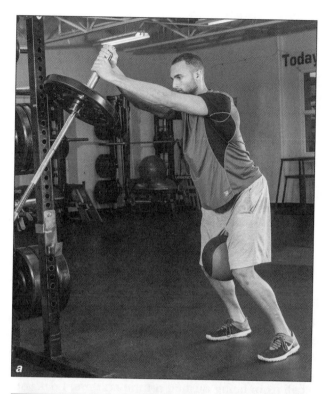

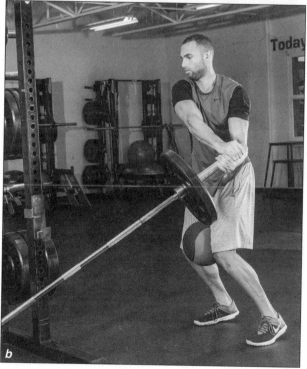

Closed Kinetic Chain (CKC) Ball Hold

This exercise can add to or replace ball hugs; the difference is the use of an athletic stance and holding the ball away from the body. This is an essential exercise for any athlete. It builds strength and stability. Developing core stability in the closed kinetic chain is a crucial step to linking your core with posture and building the core musculature to contribute to whole-body strength and movement drills.

Setup

Get into an athletic-ready stance with your feet shoulder-width apart and your ankles, knees, and hips slightly flexed. Hold a stability ball in front of you at chest height with the arms almost fully extended and hands pressing in against the sides of the ball. Set the shoulders and middle back by pulling the shoulder blades up, back, and down so that your chest is up and out. Squeezing the stability ball will help to stabilize the shoulder blades. Do not let the stability ball touch the torso.

Movement

A training partner or coach applies strong three-second pushes, alternating directly to the left and right. Maintain a contracted core, middle back, hips, and lower body. Own your position, trying to prevent your partner from moving the ball from the starting position. Think of anchoring this position, being strong to prevent the ball from being pushed off the midline. Lock your rib cage onto your hips to prevent any rotation through the trunk or flexion and extension.

Tips and Progressions

- The push is timed at three seconds to give you time to figure out what muscles to activate to counteract the push and achieve strong muscle contractions.
- Partners should not be shy about applying force. If the exerciser shows too much rotation, ease up. If the exerciser is anchored in, add more force.
- To increase difficulty, apply more force or hold the ball farther from the body, which increases the lever length from the ball to the midline.
- You can also begin to vary the direction of push, adding diagonal and vertical push patterns.
- After a set number of workouts with steady pushes, decrease the length of each push while increasing the sequence pace, applying fast repetitive strikes (fast repeats) from various directions.
- When you are no longer challenged, progress by closing the eyes.

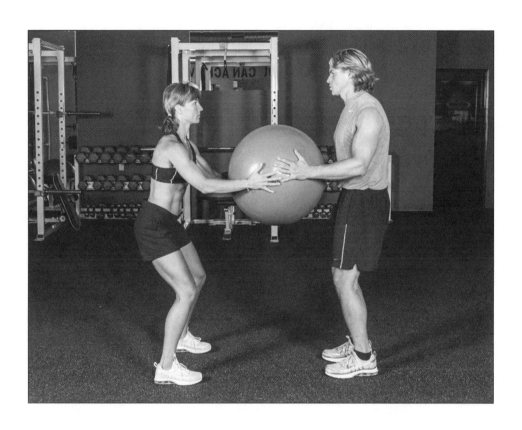

Lateral-Jump Ball Hold

Lateral-jump ball hold is similar in principle to the CKC ball hold. This exercise incorporates lateral movement mechanics with CKC core stability, linking the core to lateral deceleration and balance.

Setup

You need enough space for two athletes to jump side to side. Begin by getting into an athletic-ready stance with your feet shoulder-width apart and with your ankles, knees, and hips slightly flexed. Hold the stability ball in front of you at chest height with arms almost fully extended, hands pressing in against the sides of the ball. Set the shoulders and middle back by pulling the shoulder blades up, back, and down so that your chest is up and out. Squeezing the stability ball will help to stabilize the shoulder blades. Do not let the ball touch the torso.

Movement

To begin the exercise, preload the legs and jump off laterally 2 feet (61 cm) to your left. Land softly and absorb the landing by engaging your core and triple-flexing your ankles, knees, and hips. Immediately upon landing, have your partner or coach apply a three-second push to the ball, pushing from the inside. Think of land–contract–hold. Keep your shoulders stabilized and chest up to prevent any movement to the ball and any breakdown in posture. Repeat in the opposite direction, and alternate jumping left and right for 12 reps total.

Tips and Progressions

- When first trying the exercise, start by jumping small distances while your partner delays the push, letting you land and stabilize your posture before pushing on the ball.
- Progress by jumping greater distances, increasing the lateral loading.
- Next, your partner pushes as soon as you touch the floor from your lateral jump. To land safely, secure a positive angle, planting the outside foot out past the hips. Dorsiflex, pulling the toe up, to create a heel lock before hitting the floor, which helps prevent inversion sprains.
- To impose varied overload on the body, you can also use a DSL stability ball. When you land the lateral jump, the load inside the ball will shift so that your core also has to brace for the impact while the shoulders carry the weighted ball against gravity.

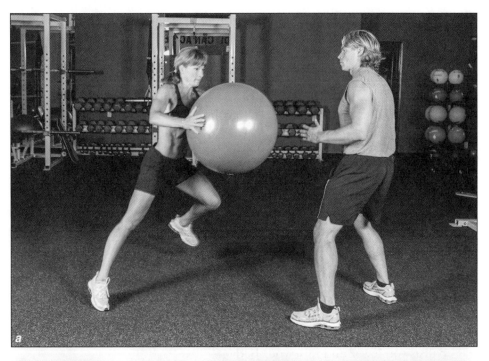

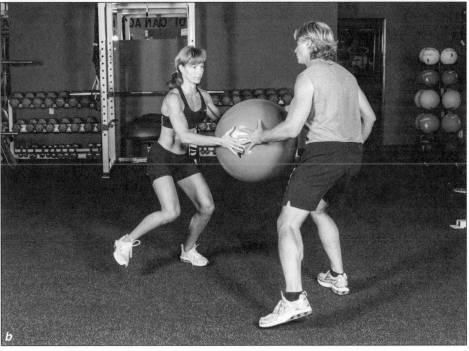

Balance Push-Up

This exercise activates all of the upper-body and core muscle groups for stabilization throughout the exercise. It is a great way to overload the muscles without loading up Olympic weights.

Setup

Standing behind the ball, place your hands on the ball at shoulder width. Shuffle your feet back until your chest is over the ball and you are supported on your toes.

Movement

Bend at the elbows to lower your chest to the ball, slowly lowering to 90 degrees at the elbows. Maintain a strongly contracted core; do not let your hips relax and sag. Hold for two seconds at the bottom. Keep your shoulders and hips square.

Finish

Extend your arms to bring your upper body back to the setup position.

Tips and Progressions

- In the push-up position, lift one foot off the floor and work to balance as you lower and push up.
- At the setup stage, place your hands on the side of the ball. Press into the ball as you lower and raise your body.

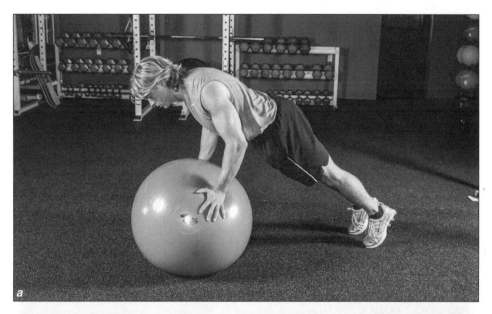

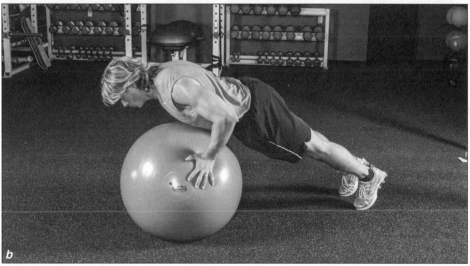

Reverse Balance Push-Up

An elevated foot placement moves more of the load to your upper body and requires more core and hip stability. We recommend this exercise in combination with balance push-ups.

Setup

Standing behind the ball, crouch down and place your abdominals on top of the ball. Roll forward until your hands reach the floor in front of the ball. Walk your hands out until only your feet remain on top of the ball. Contract the core to hold a strong link—your body should be in a straight and firm line from feet to head.

Movement

As you bend at the elbows to lower your chest to the floor, maintain your balance on the ball. Keep your torso facing square to the floor.

Finish

Hold for one second at the bottom, and then extend your arms to bring your upper body back to the setup position.

Tips and Progressions

- Once in the setup position, have a spotter position a balance board under your hands to produce dual instability.
- As you lower into the push-up, you must keep your feet balanced on the ball while also balancing your arms on the board.
- Your core must be strongly contracted to link the body together from its positions of instability.

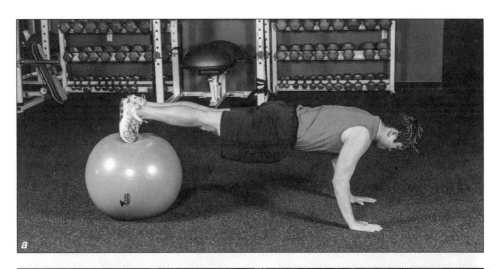

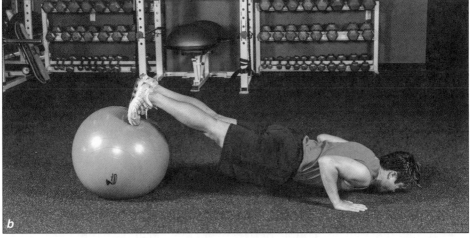

Up Up, Down Down

This is an excellent exercise for upper-body stability, posterior deltoid strength, arm strength, and trunk and pelvic stability.

Setup

Begin by getting into a prone plank position on the ball with your elbows shoulder-width apart and bent at 90 degrees. Your forearms should be directly on top of the ball. Your feet should be a little wider than shoulder-width apart, and your core is engaged so that your ankles, knees, hips, and shoulders are all in alignment. Engage your core and shoulder stabilizers.

Movement

Lead with the right arm by picking up your right arm and placing your right hand on the ball. Now push up and extend your elbow so that it is fully extended. Immediately after, lift your left elbow off and quickly place your left hand where your left elbow was. While doing this movement, try to keep your hips from rotating side to side.

Middle Position

In the middle position you should be in a prone plank position with your hands on the ball. Your core musculature is engaged to prevent the low back from sagging.

Finish

Engage your core again, and reverse the movement that got you up there. Pick up your right arm, and then place your right elbow where your hand was by using your left arm to lower yourself with control. Lift your left hand off and place your left elbow where your left hand was. Repeat for desired amount of reps. Be sure to do the same in leading the movement with your left arm.

Tips and Progressions

- It sometimes takes a couple of tries to get the feel and rhythm necessary to do the exercise correctly. For this exercise you may want to have a spotter or place the ball against a dumbbell for more stability.
- For a progression, narrow your base of support by bringing your feet closer together.
- Greater challenge comes with slowing the movement overall, with longer loading phases before adding the next movement.
- If you cannot stabilize the one-arm transitions, a DSL stability ball will provide a more stable base from which to attempt the exercise.

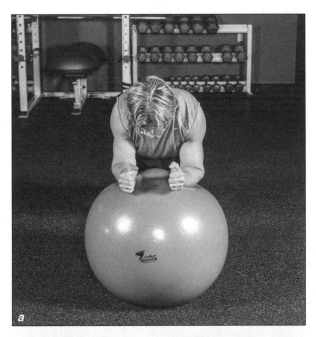

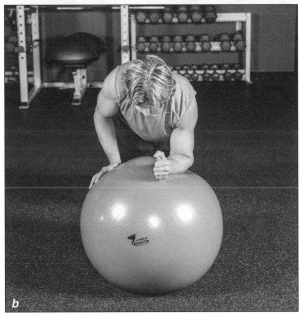

Kneeling Hold and Clock

Every exercise of every kind can be assessed in terms of a ratio of risk to benefit. For example, we do not allow our clients to stand on the ball. Although a few are capable, the risk of a substantial fall and injury is high. Part of the assessment is the exit strategy if things don't go right. There are half-balls called BOSU Balance Trainers with hundreds of standing exercises and a simple step-off exit strategy. With stability balls, we go as far as kneeling on them. Your center of mass remains close to the ball, and to exit, the feet easily slide off the ball and onto the floor. Kneeling holds and clock movements are great for grading force production in different directions and refining control of the hips and abdominals.

Setup

To get up on the ball, place your hands and then knees on the front top part of the ball. Roll forward as you release the hands. Use a narrow leg position and elevate through the rib cage for a tall postural position. Arms can be flexed at your sides, neutral.

On your first attempts at this exercise, have a spotter stand in front of you, one arm flexed. Hold the spotter's forearm to help you get up on the ball and stabilize. Gradually soften your grip on the spotter's arm. The front spotter position is easiest for you to hold and prevents you from coming off the ball forward. The other three exit options—back, to the left, and to the right—are easier for getting a foot down on the floor. Use a wider leg placement to allow adductors to squeeze into the ball to assist in balancing, and keep your hips close to your ankles, lowering your center of mass.

Movement

In your first few sets with this exercise, strive to stay on top of the ball, reacting with any necessary corrective responses to deviations in balance. It will mirror a golf swing—just when you think you have it, it becomes difficult again. Use strong bracing and minor adjustments to return the ball to the setup position, weight centered on top.

Tips and Progressions

- If you find it difficult to stay on top of the ball, select a DSL stability ball, which will decrease the instability and help you succeed at the kneeling hold.

- At the other end of the continuum, to advance the drill, purposefully shift your center of mass on the ball, which forces you to contract the correct muscles to the correct degree to return to a centered position. Start with one-inch shifts, shifting to a 3 o'clock position, then 6 o'clock, 9 o'clock, and 12 o'clock. Learn to grade the amount of force you generate so you do not overadjust. On the sideways movements to 3 o'clock and 9 o'clock, gradually increase the amount of displacement until you are striving to find and hold a finish position with one leg on top of the ball, the other leg rolled off to the side as in figure *b*, still alternating from side to side without placing a foot on the floor. This places additional demands on hip strength and control, which are essential for single-leg movements.

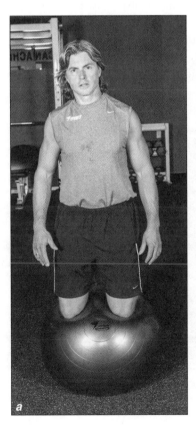
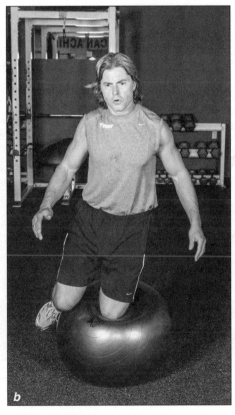

Seated Humpty Dumpty

Have fun with this one! This is a great warm-up exercise that stimulates core strength and responsiveness.

Setup

Begin by sitting up straight on a stability ball with the core muscles engaged. Find a balance point where you can lift your feet a few inches off the floor. To prevent overuse of the hip flexors while in this position, slightly lean back so the angle at the hips is 90 degrees or greater.

Movement

Between two or more people sitting on stability balls, pass a weighted ball back and forth. Do not let the feet touch the floor.

Tips and Progressions

- This is a great icebreaker exercise and can easily be turned into a game. Have fun with this—count the number of successful passes, count how long you can go before someone's foot touches down or how many passes you can get in a time frame, or add a few more medicine balls into the mix.

- You can further progress the exercise by using heavier balls, increasing the distance between the throws, or passing farther from the midline (but still in reach).

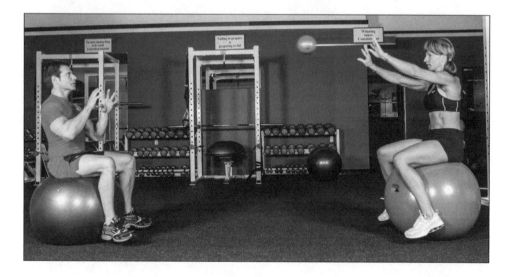

Dual-Ball Survival Rollout

This exercise is a fun and interesting challenge. Less attention is focused on body technique; rather, you will discover the right mechanics as you explore how to stay on the balls. This generates very thorough activation of the musculature through the shoulders, back, abdominals, and hips, all of which must work extremely hard to complete each rep. You will need to handle the load of your body weight and prevent sideways movement of the ball, with reactive muscle contractions to correct losses of balance.

Setup
Select two different-sized balls and set them about 6 inches (15 cm) apart. Set the heels of your hands on the top outside of the front 65-centimeter ball while you mount the knees on the back 55-centimeter ball. Establish a kneeling position, hips low, hands on the front ball, and set the midback.

Movement
Shift some of your weight onto the hands and work to hold this position without exiting the balls. React to any deviations in balance by pulling back to a centered position.

Tips and Progressions
- After you learn how to stay up on the two balls with fewer movement deviations, progress to a dual-ball rollout where you extend the arms and legs to create more separation between the balls. Start by moving both balls 1 inch (2.5 cm) and return to the setup position.
- Progress over a set number of workouts to longer extension, moving the balls as far apart as possible, as shown in the photo.
- If you reach a distance that is uncomfortable on the lumbar spine, shorten the distance you will work, potentially reverting to the static survival hold position. Also add supplemental supine bridge and prone extension exercises to prepare the back to handle greater challenges.

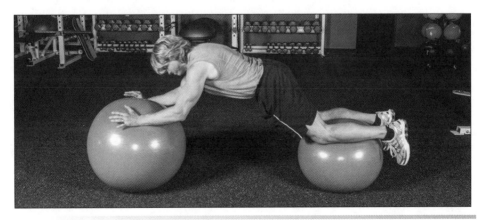

Kneeling Medicine Ball Catch

This exercise requires that a dynamic load be caught in an unstable position. By removing the eccentric action of the legs, the entire responsibility to stabilize is left to the core.

Setup

To get up on the ball, place your hands and then knees on the front top part of the ball. Roll forward as you release the hands. Use a narrow leg position and elevate through the rib cage for a tall postural position. Draw in and brace the core and set the middle back. Extend the arms out at chest level. Your coach or partner positions about 6 feet (1.8 m) away, directly in front of you.

Movement

Stay as solid as possible on top of the ball, making continuous minor adjustments to any deviations in balance. The coach begins passing the ball directly down the midline, straight to your hands. Flex at the elbows to cushion the catch while you contract through the core, glutes, and adductors to keep your weight centered on the ball. When you have secured a stable position, pass the ball back to the coach, prepare to break momentum after ball release, and stay on top of the ball.

Tips and Progressions

- If this exercise is not manageable, replace it with two exercises: kneeling hold and clock along with medicine ball shoulder-to-shoulder pass (this chapter and chapter 8, respectively). After perfecting the advanced progressions in both of those exercises, try the kneeling medicine ball catch again.

- To work on progressive overload, the coach can deliver passes outside the midline so you catch in front of one shoulder, making stabilization on top of the ball more difficult.

- Next, the coach positions off to one side to distribute cross-body passes that you catch with two hands in front of the body, allowing slight rotation while maintaining control.

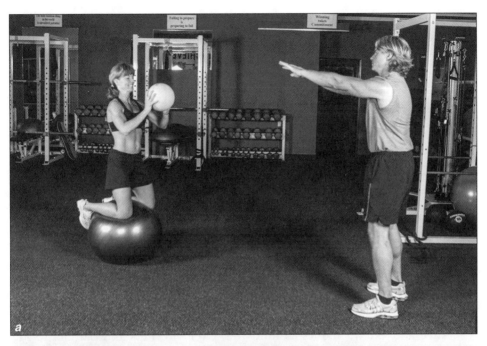

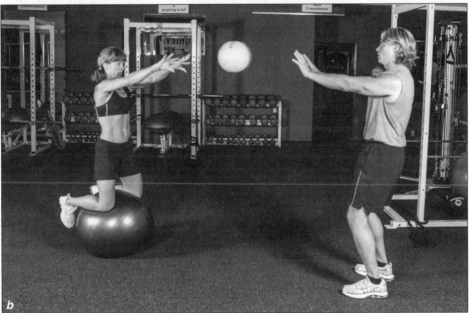

Progressive Tabletop

This exercise uses a four-point stance to activate the core, integrating instability and reduced base of support to heighten the activation of muscles.

Setup

In a standing position, place your knees in contact with the ball; position your hands on top of the ball. Load your weight onto the hands as you shift your weight forward, bringing the feet off the floor. When in place with a four-point stance, knees are on top of the ball and hands are slightly forward. Draw in and brace your core.

Movement

Contract your glutes, hips, abdominals, back, and shoulders to anchor this position, making minor adjustments to correct any deviations in balance. Focus on retaining a set middle-back position, holding and correcting movement without hunching your shoulders. Lift one arm, holding it straight out parallel to the trunk. Alternate arms.

Tips and Progressions

- Enhance core strength by trying the same maneuver with one leg. Lift a knee and extend the leg behind you, level with hips and parallel to the floor. Glutes will fire aggressively and likewise the shoulders and lats will work hard to hold the position on the ball.

- Once you can hold an extended leg with solid coordination for 20 seconds, you are ready to progress to opposite arm and leg, lifting one arm up and also lifting the opposite leg as shown in figure b.

- If you weren't able to achieve the original tabletop on the ball, adopt the progressions listed previously (lift arm, progress to leg, progress to opposite arm or leg), but do them on a mat on the floor. This will help you build the required strength to eventually get back up on the ball into a tabletop position.

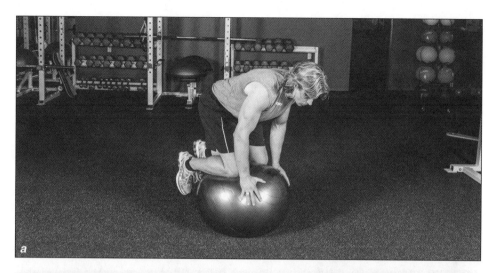

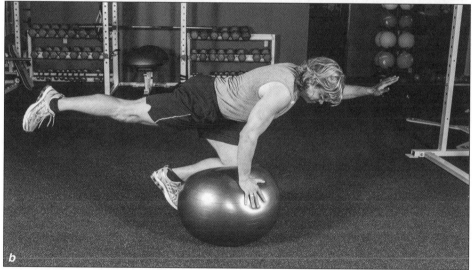

Kneeling Rollout

This is an excellent exercise for overloading the core through a full range of motion with a natural rolling motion. Rollouts produce eccentric elongation as well as isometric contraction. This exercise also works the chest, back, shoulders, and triceps muscle groups.

Setup

Kneel in front of a ball and produce a pelvic tilt, moving your glutes forward and drawing in your navel toward your spine. Place your hands on top of the ball and bring your feet off the floor. This allows your knees to become the pivot point. Walk your hands out on the ball, moving the ball and your arms away from your body. Once you feel your abdominals beginning to work, you have reached your starting position.

Movement

Your hands will remain stationary on the ball. Pivot on your knees and bring your torso and hips forward as the ball rolls away from your knees. Keep moving until your chest drops down. Keep your chest upright as much as possible, avoiding the Superman pose. If you feel any strain in your lower back, make sure you are not in the Superman pose. If your back discomfort remains, return to the setup stage and check your pelvic tilt.

Finish

Hold at the far reach for two seconds, then roll back into the starting position.

Tips and Progressions

- In the extended rollout position, rather than holding stationary for two seconds, move the ball outside of your midline to place additional demands on the core muscles. Try a figure-eight pattern or a side-to-side movement aiming to move your right hand in front of your left shoulder (and left hand to right shoulder on the reverse), or select a word to spell. For example, in the far extended position, move the ball to spell each letter in power; that completes one rep before you return to the setup position.

- Progress to a single-arm rollout. Keep the ball positioned down your midline, and remove one hand to perform one-arm kneeling rollouts.

- Complete single-arm kneeling rollouts with the ball positioned outside of midline, more in line with your active arm. This produces additional loading on the shoulder, triceps, and abdominals. Stabilizing muscles have to work harder to prevent hip and torso rotation.

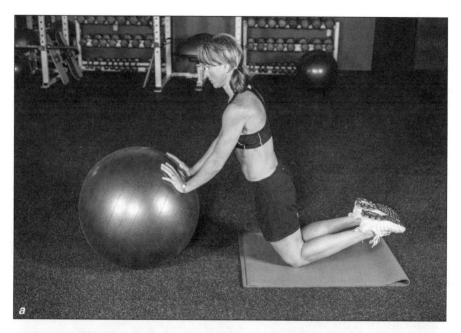

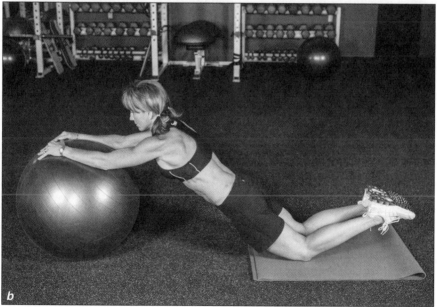

Full-Body Multijoint Medicine Ball Pass

This exercise produces sequential full-body power as well as anaerobic conditioning.

Setup

Stand facing your partner, about six paces apart. Keep your feet shoulder-width apart, knees slightly flexed, and abdominals contracted.

Movement

Before you pass the ball, squat down and touch the ball to the floor. The pass begins from this position. Maintain a good squat position, chest up and back in a safe position. The throw begins with the legs and transfers through the hips and on to the upper body. The force–ground relationship is important here, because you will need to finish with a powerful leg extension, jumping right off the floor.

Remember the desired ball direction is forward, not just up, so you must drive up and out (forward) to direct the force in the intended direction.

Finish

Your partner should not attempt to catch this long-distance pass. Through trial and error, your partner will be positioned to allow the ball to land on the floor and catch it on the bounce, which is safer and easier on the body. After receiving the ball, your partner squats and touches the ball to the floor before driving up and forward with the entire body to pass a maximal distance. Every pass is a best effort. You try to work your partner backward, throwing a longer distance with all of your power.

Tips and Progressions

- Get twisted lateral two-ball pass: This drill uses the same throw technique. Both partners start with a medicine ball at opposite sides of the drill course. On "Go," both throw for maximal distance. Then immediately begin a quick lateral shuffle to the other side, where you will pick up your partner's ball and throw it back, right from the floor with a full-body squat throw.

- Continue throwing for maximal distance and shuffling at maximal speed for 30 seconds. As your anaerobic conditioning improves, increase the drill time. The intensity of this drill is 110 percent.

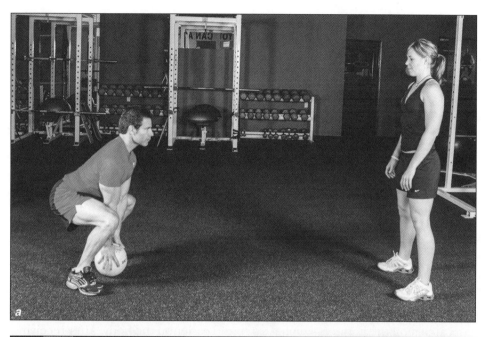

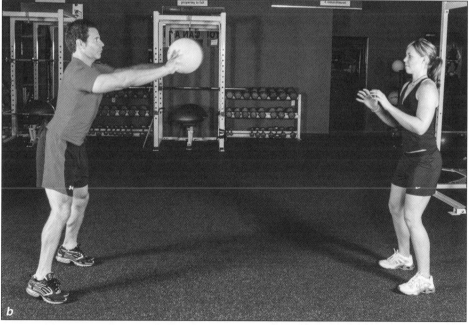

Bridge Perturbation

From a bridge position, a second ball is used for a variety of dynamic stabilizing load movements to foster reactive muscle capabilities through the eccentric–concentric responses.

Setup

Assume a supine bridge position on top of a ball. Feet are in a narrow stance, hips up strong, core set. Hold a DSL stability ball up over the chest, arms extended.

Movement

1. Keeping the arms close to full extension, complete small and large circles with fluid, consistent movement so you can hear the DSL flow around the ball.

2. Shift the DSL stability ball side to side, moving wider and faster until you accommodate with torso rotation. Listen for the impact of the DSL traveling across the ball, which you will also feel as you brace for the impact of the DSL.

3. Complete a sit-up pattern. Sit up and extend the arms in front of your chest. Sit back down into the supine bridge position, arms out over head. Again, absorb the force of the DSL as it shifts across to the other side of the ball at each end range of motion.

Tips and Progressions

- Begin with smaller ranges of motion and regress by keeping the ball closer to your torso.
- Progress by adding more load to the ball.

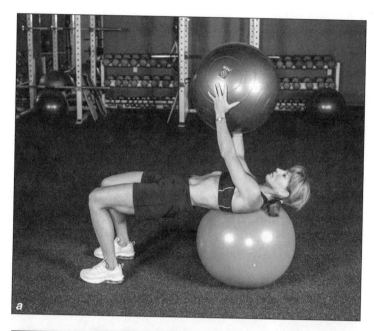

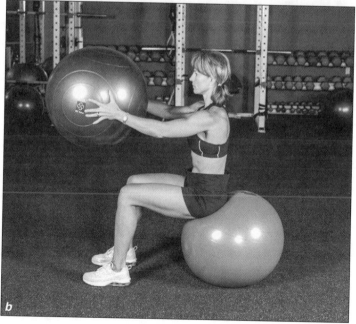

Supine Bridge Ball Hold

The supine bridge is one of the foundational ball positions that so many exercises build from, developing the deep core musculature plus obliques, shoulders, pecs, low back, glutes, and hamstrings.

Setup

Begin in bridge position with feet flat on the floor and spaced hip-width apart. Knees are at 90 degrees, and head and shoulders are fully supported on the stability ball. Arms are extended, holding a medicine ball directly above the chest. Elbows are bent slightly but locked in position. Keep the hips up and core engaged.

Movement

Your partner stands behind your head to apply three-second pushes on the medicine ball, alternating left and right. Your goal is to keep the core locked in and not allow any movement in the arms or core. On the second set, shift to rapid-fire pushes, delivering a strong, quick push immediately followed by a push in the opposite direction, continuing for 20 seconds.

Tips and Progressions

- If the medicine ball deviates far outside the midline, ease up on the push.
- Most partners err by pushing too lightly. Push with enough force so that your partner has to struggle to maintain the medicine ball position.
- Athletes who are extremely strong in the bridge position can also be challenged by
  1. bringing the feet closer together to lessen the base of support,
  2. closing the eyes, or
  3. varying the direction of the medicine ball push (left, right, forward, back, diagonal).

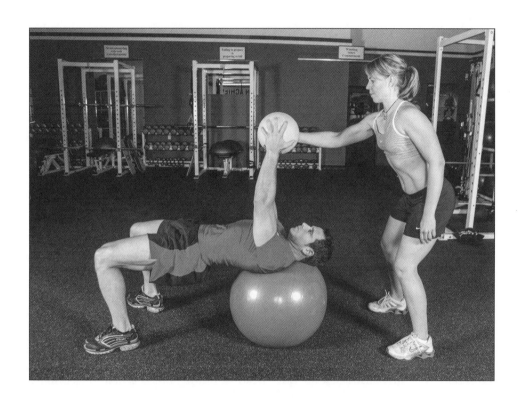

Squat to Supine to Sit-Up

In this integrated exercise, you work a squat pattern and transition to supine, where you complete a sit-up.

Setup

Begin with your DSL stability ball in neutral position (label up). The DSL stability ball has circle markings that you can use as a reference point to complete the supine portion without ball movement and to define a spot to aim for that will help you avoid falling off the ball.

Standing with your back toward the DSL stability ball, squat down so that your glutes touch at about the outer edge of the large top circle. Sit down on the top front side of the DSL stability ball, and position the feet so that the upper legs are parallel to the floor with the feet in a shoulder-width stance. You might have to adjust the distance you are standing from the ball to find the correct position.

Movement

Without any arm swing, come up to a standing position, then squat back down until the glutes rest back on the top front side of the ball. Lower the torso under control into a supine bridge position. Lift one leg off the floor and hold for three seconds; repeat with other leg.

Finish

With both feet on the floor, slowly lift your torso off the ball, segment by segment, rising up to a seated position before standing.

Tips and Progressions

- The ball does not roll during this exercise. It should remain in a neutral position, which you can check by starting the exercise with the logo at the top.
- Repeat the sequence for a desired rep count; however, as you close in on the finishing reps, fatigue may determine that you eliminate the leg-lift portion so you can effectively continue with the squat to sit-up and finish strong.

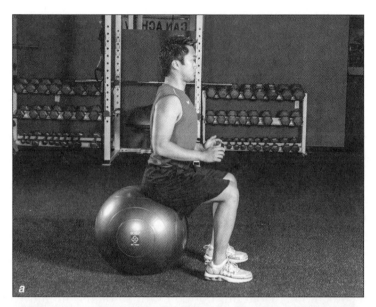

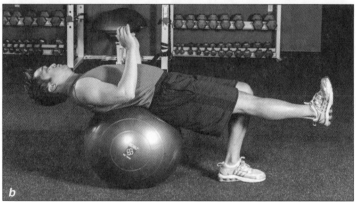

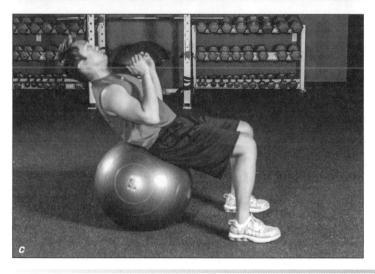

Stability Ball Static Lateral Crunch With Medicine Ball Punch-Out

This is a great combination exercise that focuses on core stabilization through the frontal and transverse planes. Challenges are presented by weight of a loaded ball and time held in the most difficult position.

Setup

At a wall, lean into the apex of the ball with your feet spread apart approximately 42 inches (~1 m). This will vary based on leg length, but ensure you feel stable and use the wall to anchor your feet. The bottom leg should be forward.

Movement

Hold a medicine ball in close to your chest and set up so you are in a lateral crunch position on the ball. Your head, shoulders, hips, and knees should form a nearly straight line. Hold this position with absolutely no movement. This is the challenge to the frontal plane.

Finish

While holding the lateral position, punch the ball out at chest level and fully extend your arms. Hold the position for 3 to 5 seconds and return to your chest.

Tips and Progressions

- This is an advanced exercise that may require no medicine ball to start. Try using just your arms.
- If you can complete 8 to 10 reps with a 3- to 5-second hold, progress to a small medicine ball and progress from there.

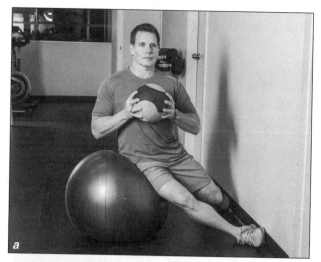

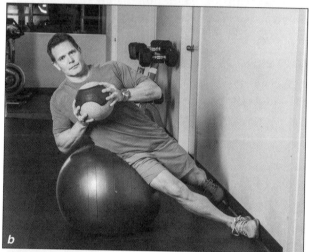

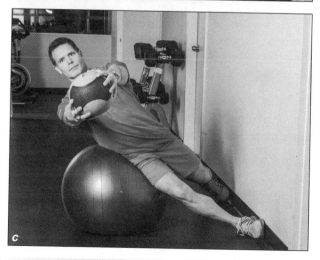

Step and Push Back

This power exercise loads the core and trains sequential firing among the legs, hips, abdominals, and upper extremities.

Setup

Stand with feet at shoulder width, facing your partner. Assume an athletic-ready position. Your partner holds a small medicine ball.

Movement

Your partner delivers a pass directly to one shoulder. As the ball approaches, step forward with one leg.

Finish

Upon making contact with the ball, immediately push the ball away from the body, straight out from your shoulder and back to your partner. Return to a ready position. Continue for a set number of reps.

Tips and Progressions

Upon making ball contact and initiating the push, remember your hips and core—the speed center—must get behind this action and assist in the force production.

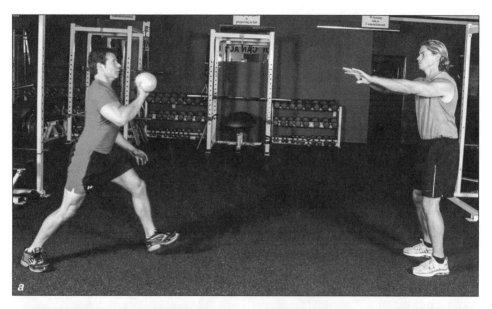

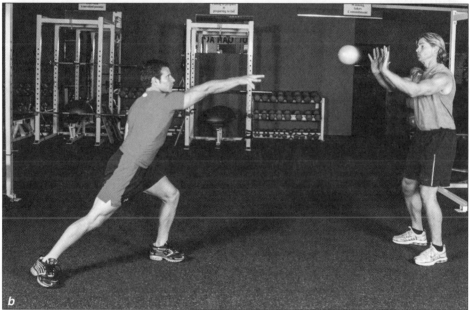

One-Leg Opposite-Arm Medicine Ball Pass

This exercise teaches you to decelerate and catch with the entire body while building posterior deltoid, pectoral, core, hip, and leg strength to catch and balance on one leg. Ultimately, body position relies heavily on core stability during all positions of the exercise.

Setup

Begin facing a partner at least 6 feet (1.8 m) apart. Each partner stands on the same single leg (for example, both stand on the left leg). Partner A holds a medicine ball at the shoulder opposite the standing support leg. Partner B presents a target with arm extended and hand open, preparing to receive the ball. Partner B will tend to set up with the hand close to the shoulder; make sure he or she has the hand out away from the body ready to receive the ball. To initiate movement, partner A preloads the leg by dropping body mass 2 inches (5 cm) before extending the leg, transferring power from the leg through the core and out through the arm.

Movement

Partner A passes the medicine ball across to partner B. Partner B receives the pass, catching by flexing the arm, braking with the core, and flexing at the knee and ankle to absorb the weight of the ball. Keep the chest up, shoulders back, and core engaged to avoid excess rotation. Before returning the pass, take time to regain balance and ensure the knee tracks in line with the toes and over the ankle. Alternate the standing leg on passes.

Tips and Progressions

- Use a slow tempo, counting 2 seconds on the concentric and eccentric phases. Pause in the middle to perfect a single-leg balanced position.
- Slow catching mechanics will prove more difficult in terms of strength, stability, and balance.
- For even greater adaptations, slow down the catch sequence and shift into a deeper leg position.
- To increase the transferability to sport skills, decrease the coupling time between the catch and pass (eccentric–concentric phases) and increase the tempo and the power of the throw.

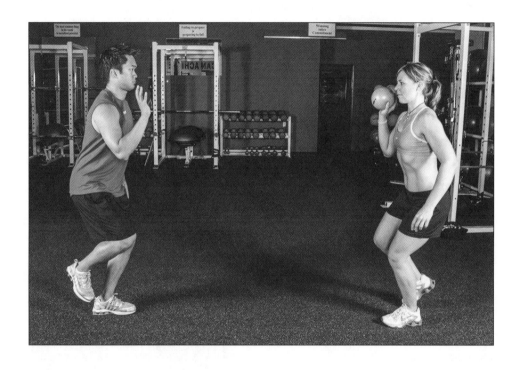

Medicine Ball Single-Leg Balance Left to Right

Left-to-right exercise produces excellent balance and proprioception responses while overloading the speed center. The deep abdominal wall and core muscles contribute through eccentric loading, stabilization, and concentric action. The single-leg stance accelerates the demands on the speed center. You will feel every muscle working from toes to abdominals.

Setup

Stand on one leg with knee slightly flexed. Set the abdominals and focus on balance. Hold the ball with two hands in front of your body.

Movement

Move the ball over to the left side of your body, but do not rotate the torso. The torso and shoulders should remain square, facing straight forward. Move the ball back across the body and over to the right side of the body.

Finish

Continue to move the ball alternately from the left to right sides of your body, reacting to the changing load position by contracting the abs, hips, and legs. Your degree of knee flexion will adjust appropriately to counterbalance the shifting load positioning.

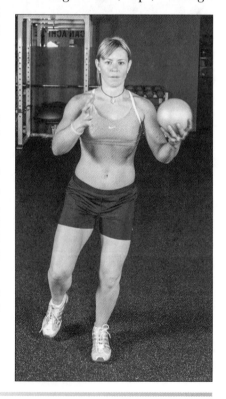

Tips and Progressions

- Increase the speed of movement.
- Move the ball farther away from the body, farther off to the side, and farther in front of the body upon rotation.
- Toss the ball from the left hand to the right hand as shown in the photo. Catch and absorb with the arm, core, and leg. This increases the balance challenge and also increases the load on the abdominals. This is an excellent abdominal exercise.
- Rapid-fire toss: Move the ball from the left hand to the right hand as quickly as possible.

CHAPTER 5

CORE ROTATION

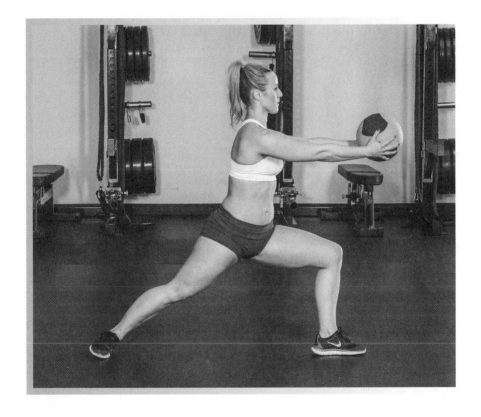

Russian Twist

The Russian twist is an excellent exercise for integrating static extension and rotational trunk movement. Movement of this nature occurs in many sport situations, including football, rugby, hockey, and tennis.

Setup

Sitting on a ball, walk forward, allowing the ball to roll underneath you. Keep walking out until your head and shoulders are supported by the ball. Arms should be extended over your chest, your abdominals set, and your core parallel to the floor.

Movement

Begin by rotating all the way to one side. Ensure rotation is initiated by the core. Many first-timers to the Russian twist will initiate rotation from the shoulder. It is also important to keep your eyes on your hands, enhancing the total core rotation as you move.

Finish

As you reach your end range, change direction and then begin moving in the opposite direction.

Tips and Progressions

- Hold a medicine ball or dumbbell in hand.
- By setting up in front of an adjustable cable, you will obtain greater loading in both directions as a result of the constant loading from the cable.

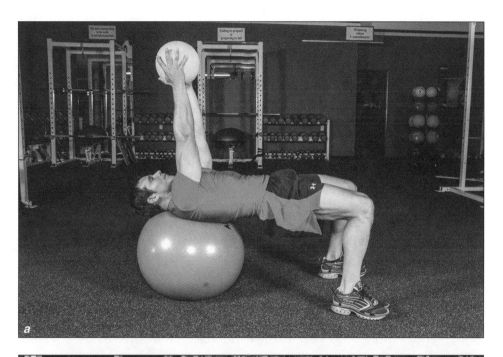

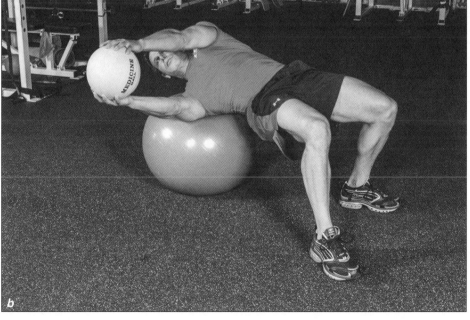

Supine Bridge With Cross-Body Pass

The diagonal firing patterns associated with the catch–throw phase link the shoulder and opposite hip with a core pattern that is transferable to many activities.

Setup

Partner A is in a supine bridge position: shoulders on the ball, neck supported and neutral, hips up, and feet hip-width apart and firmly planted on the floor. Feet should be positioned far enough out so the knee joint is at 90 degrees and not shooting out over the toes. With a medicine ball in the hands, arms are extended up in line with the chest. Partner B stands to the right of partner A about 5 feet (1.5 m) away in a good athletic stance, ready to give and receive the medicine ball passes.

Start Position

Partner A rotates from the core onto the left shoulder, keeping the hips squared and feet planted, dropping the hands (with medicine ball) off to the left side in line with the shoulders.

Movement

Partner A rotates from the left shoulder around to the right, releasing the ball to partner B. Partner A decelerates the rotational movement to the right so that partner A can receive the pass back from partner B and return to the start position. Repeat the exercise going from the right to the left.

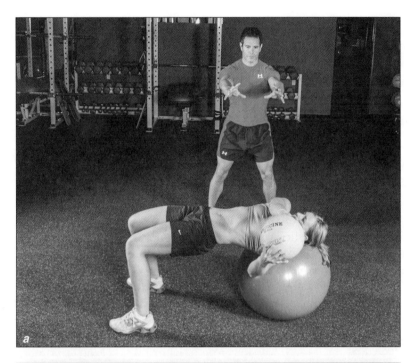

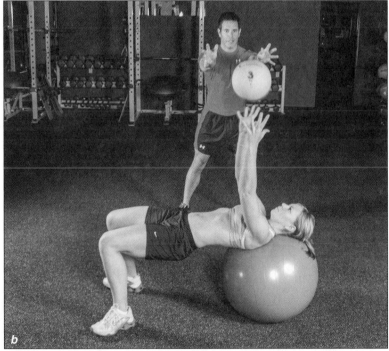

Over-the-Shoulder Throw

This exercise builds full-body power and torso rotation and produces sequential muscle firing for a smooth multijoint throw. Multijoint power in a closed kinetic chain through a transverse plane applies to many sports and activities.

Setup

Stand facing away from a partner, about two paces apart. Keep your feet shoulder-width apart, knees well flexed, and abdominals contracted. Your partner is facing you (looking at your back), one step to the right.

Movement

Before you throw the ball, squat down and rotate to bring the ball in front of your right shin. The throw initiates from this position. Be sure to use a squat movement, dropping your hips to lower the ball to shin height so there is not excessive forward trunk flexion. The throw begins at the foot, transfers through your right leg, and transfers through the hips and torso and on to the upper body.

Remember the desired ball direction is behind to your partner, not just up, so you must rotate through the torso and follow through behind you to direct the ball from above your left shoulder to your partner, who is standing behind you and off to your right.

Finish

Your partner catches the ball and rolls it back to your right side, where you can pick it up and move into the sequential throw technique. Repeat for the desired number of repetitions, then repeat the exercise throwing over the opposite (right) shoulder. Your partner will change his position, staying two paces behind you but shifting to your left side.

Tips and Progressions

- After you release the throw, keep your hands up above your shoulders.
- Your partner will catch your throw and return a gentle pass into your hands, where you catch it above your shoulders, rotate, and squat to the opposite side.
- Then thrust upward to throw the ball back over the same shoulder.

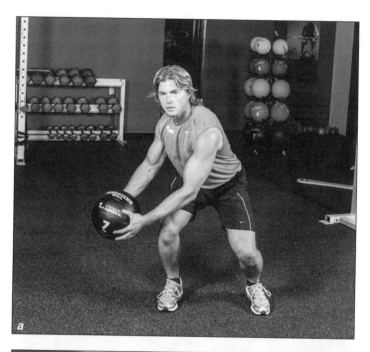

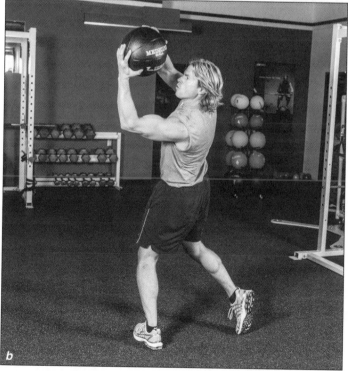

Twister

This exercise places a weight at the end of a lever arm to increase the demands of the torso to stabilize and direct movement.

Setup

Lie on the floor in a supine position with your arms straight out to the sides. Make sure you achieve a solid pelvic tilt. Set the abdominals before lifting the legs into the air. Legs are together and flexed to 90 degrees. Place a small medicine ball between your knees. Press inward to hold the ball in place and activate your adductors and hip musculature.

Movement

Slowly lower the knees under control, off to the right side. Shoulders and back must remain flat on the floor.

Finish

Lift the legs back up over your hips (still flexed) and onward to the left side. Lower to the left. Stop and return. Continue for desired number of reps or until you lose neutral torso supine position.

Tips and Progressions

- Complete the same sequence with more speed. Drop legs to the left, and activate muscles to decelerate and stop before touching the floor. Return across the body to the opposite side.

- Position the legs into a straight position over the body and position the ball between the ankles to increase the lever arm and place the loading farther out on the lever.

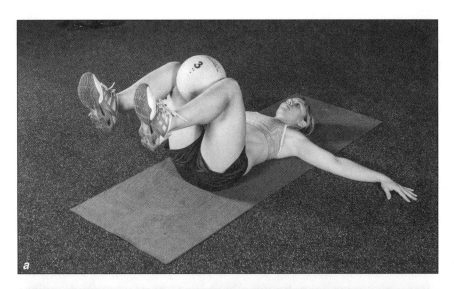

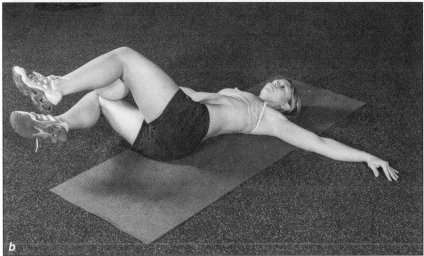

Supine Rotator Scissors

Supine scissors will place a great challenge on the abdominals from a static perspective.

Setup

Lying on the floor, place a ball between your feet and ankles; squeeze. Place your hands under your back at the L3 (midlumbar) level of your spine, engage your core, and maintain the pressure you feel on your hands.

Movement

Begin by raising your feet and the ball so to create a 45-degree angle at your hips. While squeezing the ball, rotate at your hips so that one foot rotates over the other.

Finish

Return to the start position and rotate to the opposite side.

Tips and Progressions

- If you do not have the shoulder flexibility to place your hands under your low back, leave them by your sides, and consciously think about pressing your spine into the floor.
- You can progress this movement by raising and lowering the legs and ball after each rotation.

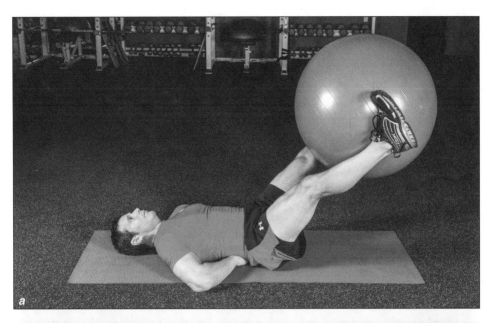

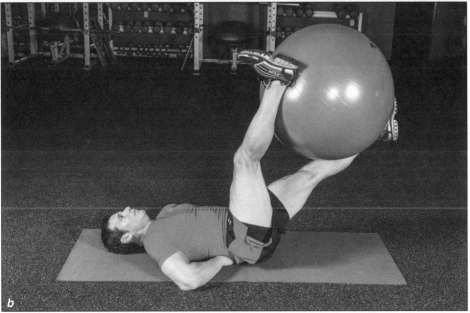

Prone Twist

The prone twist combines a challenge in both the sagittal and transverse planes. This movement ties in the hips, shoulders, and core.

Setup

Begin with the ball under your abdomen and hands on the floor in a push-up position. Walk your hands forward so the ball begins to roll toward your feet. At this point, widen your feet over the ball, and squeeze. Your shoulders and core must be firing before you initiate the movement.

Movement

Laterally roll the ball to one side by rotating your hips.

Finish

Hold end range for a second, then return and rotate to the opposite side.

Tips and Progressions

- Most errors in the prone twist occur as you begin the movement. What you need to avoid is a drop in the low back.
- By keeping your core engaged, you will feel the work of the lower portion of your abdominals.
- The low back should be held in a neutral position or should be slightly kyphotic (rounded).

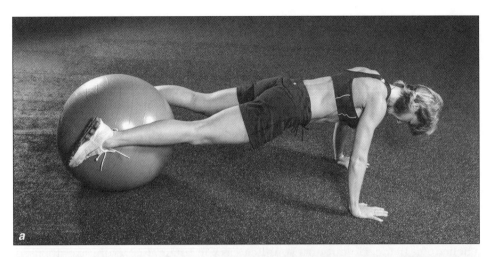

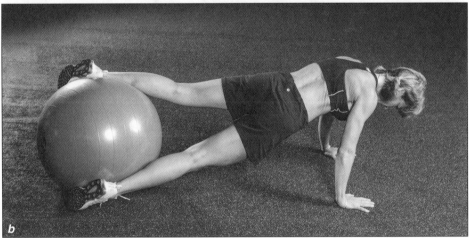

Goldy's Static Lateral Helicopter

The static lateral helicopter was developed as a progression from the abdominal side crunch.

Setup

Set up this movement with your feet at the base of the wall and floor. Your bottom leg should be forward and top leg braced back as you sit laterally on the ball. Placement on the ball should be so that your hips are at the apex of the ball. Core should be in a position so that there is a straight line from the ear to the shoulders, hips, and knees.

Movement

While you're holding the static lean position, your arms should be extended and level with your shoulders. Begin the movement by rotating your upper core as far as you can turn. Maintain your arm position as you rotate so your arms resemble a helicopter blade. Do not turn your head as you rotate. Keep your eyes focused straight up to the ceiling.

Finish

Complete your repetitions to one side, then repeat on the other.

Tips and Progressions

- You can increase the difficulty of this movement by holding dumbbells in each hand.
- You will find that 2 to 5 pounds (about 1 to 2 kg) will be quite challenging.

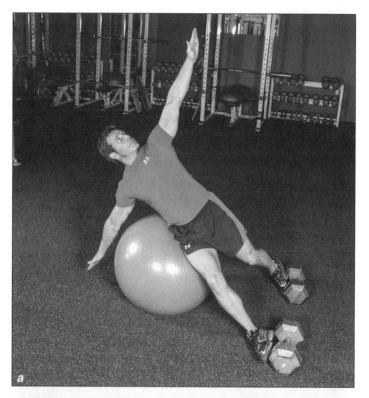

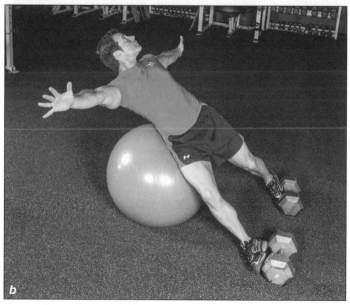

BISHOP BURTON COLLEGE

Side-to-Side Rotation Pass

This is a good warm-up exercise that gently works the legs, hips, torso, and upper body. With more powerful passes, it is a great torso rotation strength exercise, pertinent to so many sports.

Setup

Partners are four strides apart, both facing the same wall. One partner has a medicine ball. Feet are positioned shoulder-width apart, knees flexed, abdominals set, head turned to see partner.

Movement

All parts of the body work together to produce the rotation pass. Push off your outside foot, and transfer the force through the hips and into torso rotation while the arms draw the ball across your body. Release the ball with a full follow-through, aiming the ball so your partner can catch it in front of the body.

Finish

Catch the ball with a strong core to protect the lower back. Absorb the catch by flexing the knee of the outside leg, rotating the torso to the outside, and allowing the arms to travel across the body to an exaggerated position off to the side. Stop and reverse the process to return the pass to your partner.

Tips and Progressions

- Static catch: Flex the knees a little more to prepare to catch the ball in front of your body, and use the abdominals to completely brake the path of the ball.
- Catch the ball and stop its travel right in front of your body.
- Once stationary, move back into the normal catch reception movement to prepare to throw the ball back to your partner.

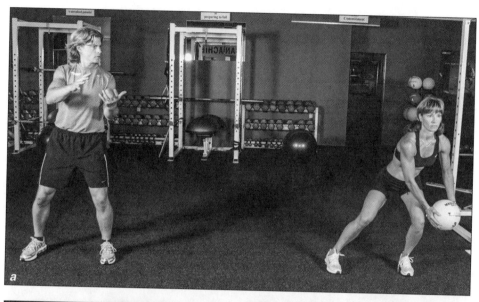

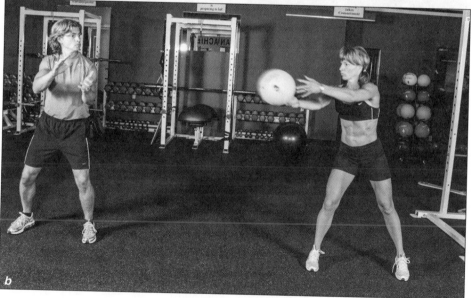

Strength Ball Prone Thoracic Rotation

From a perspective of spinal health, thoracic rotation is an area that many people can improve on. Mobility in this region will result in more effective movement patterns in your sport and daily activities.

Setup

Place a strength ball under your pelvis with feet and hands planted on the ground and head in a neutral position.

Movement

Take a dumbbell in one hand and stabilize yourself over the ball with your three points of contact. With a straight arm, begin to rotate your body in a rotary fashion without your pelvis breaking contact with the ball.

Finish

Rotate all the way around until you feel some tightness at the end of the range of motion. Pause in this position and return. Complete repetitions on the opposite side.

Tips and Progressions

- If you allow your pelvis to lose contact with the ball during the movement, it will negate the effect you are hoping to achieve in the thoracic area.

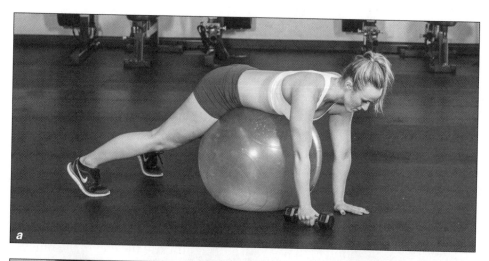

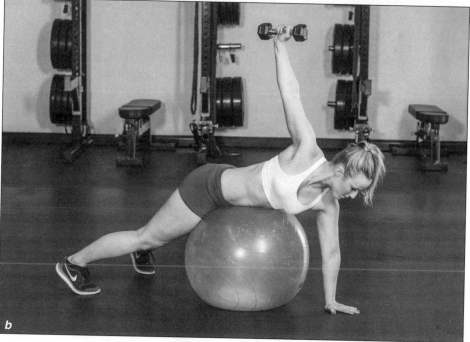

Standing Overhead Medicine Ball Rotation

This exercise focuses on full body extension while rotating in a circular fashion from the hips.

Setup

Your feet should be placed about shoulder-width apart and a medicine ball held in the hands overhead. Focus on full body extension with knees slightly bent and legs loaded into a good athletic position.

Movement

Engage your core and begin by making a circular movement while maintaining the ball overhead. Movement needs to be slow and controlled.

Finish

Complete a set amount of rotations in each direction.

Tips and Progressions

- Start with small circular movements and progress to larger movements.
- Make sure you maintain your spinal position without overextending or flexing your low back.

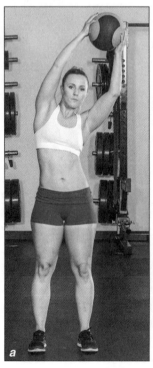 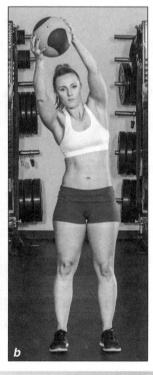

Back-to-Back Stop-and-Go

This is a great torso rotation exercise that also works the muscles eccentrically, building braking strength. Stopping and reversing direction help to overload the torso musculature.

Setup

With a partner, stand back to back, about 6 inches (15 cm) apart. Keep your feet shoulder-width apart, knees slightly flexed, and abdominals contracted.

Movement

It is important to clearly differentiate this exercise from the back-to-back 180-degree rotation pass. In the stop-and-go execution, once you pass the ball, you stay in place awaiting the ball to be returned. This helps focus the effort on a strong rotation rep and an aggressive eccentric–concentric coupling when the direction is reversed. Holding the ball away from the body, partner A rotates around to the right with speed and abruptly stops the ball off to the side, quickly returning to the left to pass the ball off to the partner. Partner B picks up the ball on the right side and immediately rotates with speed to the left. Once all the way around to the left side, partner B stops abruptly and quickly rotates back to the original (right) side to drop off the ball.

Finish

Continue this sequence for a set number of repetitions. Repeat the opposite way around.

Tips and Progressions

- Move your feet right together, and keep your knees bent.
- Move the ball farther away from your body.
- Rotate with greater speed.
- Stop more quickly.

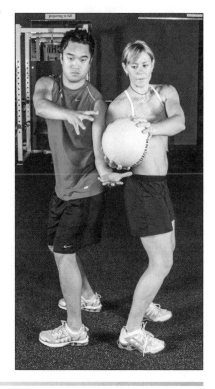

Alternating Open-Step Medicine Ball Lunge With Long-Lever Rotation

Integrating movement skills into lower-body strength, in particular how that interacts to sequence whole-body action, is a key to making gym training transfer into sport action and daily active living.

Setup

Begin facing away from your intended direction of movement in an athletic-ready position holding the medicine ball in both hands.

Movement

Pick up your left knee and externally rotate the left leg, reaching with the foot to turn and lunge 180 degrees. As you externally rotate at the hips and lunge with the leg, carry the ball as far as possible away from the torso, using the arms as long levers to produce a wide-arc movement with the hands.

Finish

Return to start position and then step to lunge to the opposite side, externally rotating at the hips and rotating the ball around to the right.

Tips and Progressions

- Maintain a slower and controlled tempo. Aim to lift the knee higher and reach the foot farther, forcing the body to stabilize and control during movement.

- Later change the progression to higher speed without sacrificing length or depth of stride or length of arm levers. Really try to push off that front lunged leg to kick it back to the start position, building more strength in the legs.

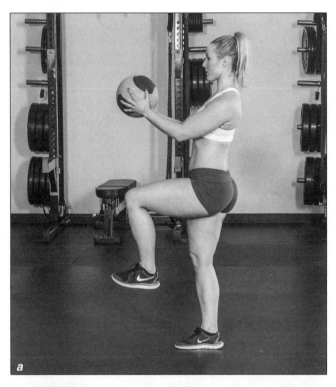

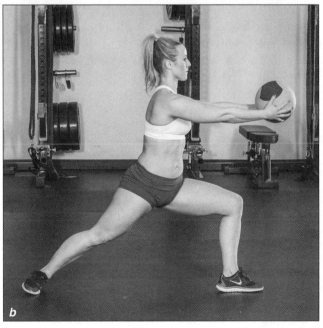

Medicine Ball Split Russian Twist

This is a movement whose prime focus is core rotation, but it also requires good static strength from the lower body because you fight gravity to maintain the position.

Setup

Get into the split position so that the front knee is directly over your foot. Lower to a position that creates a 90-degree angle at the knee joint. The rear leg should be back far enough to provide a decent stretch on the hip flexors without causing too much anterior rotation in the pelvis.

Movement

Hold the medicine ball horizontal to the floor with arms fully extended; rotate back and forth while you maintain a tall and strong core.

Finish

A single rep involves a rotation from the start position to the left and right.

Tips and Progressions

- Start with controlled rotations until the movement pattern is solid. Then increase speed and use the stretch reflex by changing direction quickly during your rotations.
- You can progress this movement by using a heavier ball, strength band, or cable. You can stress the legs more by using a weight vest.
- To open up your body, advance into a longer lunge and lower the hips deeper. To develop length and strength in the lower extremities, aim to sustain stability in this advanced static position while you twist with the medicine ball.

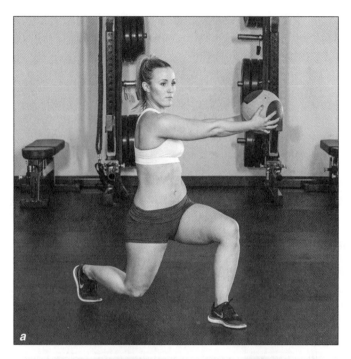

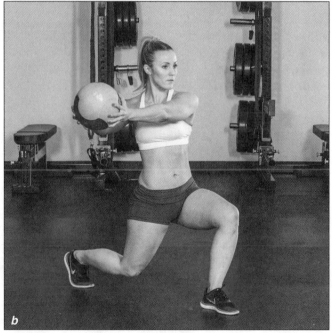

Standing Rotary Repeat

Closed kinetic chain rotary power and eccentric braking are trained through perturbations provided by the dynamic stabilizing load inside the ball. This builds strength and helps prevent sport injury.

Setup

Begin in a standing position, feet shoulder-width apart, and knees flexed. Core is set and braced; midback is set. Hold a DSL stability ball at midtorso height, hands pressing inward. Double-check for scapular retraction.

Movement

Rapidly shift the ball side to side for a 2-inch (5 cm) distance, staying close to the midline. Brake and immediately shift back to the original side. Alternate sides in quick succession. Keep the hips square as the torso rotates slightly.

Tips and Progressions

- Check your speed and force of movement with audible feedback—you should hear the DSL hitting the side of the ball as you brake at the end of each range of motion.

- Progressively increase the rotation distance until eventually you move the ball outside the torso. As the range increases and greater torso rotation is needed, allow the hips to pivot as well, linking into the core.

- As distance joins speed and force, you will be required to apply stronger deceleration to brake when the DSL strikes against the ball.

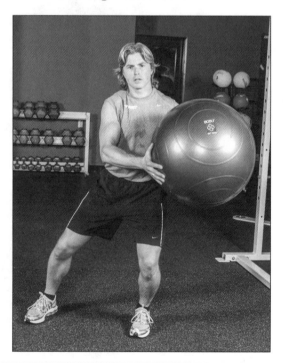

Medicine Ball Standing Twist Against Wall

This movement will assist you with increasing your rotational range of motion around the core.

Setup

In front of a wall, place your feet shoulder-width apart, approximately 6 to 8 inches (15 to 20 cm) from the wall. Your glutes should be in contact with the wall, and you can hold a medicine ball in front at midchest level. This exercise completes the prone thoracic rotation exercise as outlined earlier in this chapter.

Movement

Rotate your core from the start position so that the ball makes contact with the wall.

Finish

Come off the wall explosively and rotate to the opposite side. Again, come off the wall explosively and repeat.

Tips and Progressions

- To increase the difficulty and progress with your range of motion, you can move your body forward off the wall. By doing this, you will increase the range of motion that is required of your core to turn and get the ball to the wall.

- Once you have progressed your range of motion, you can continue to progress by wrapping the ball in a towel and completing the movement by bouncing the ball hard off the wall.

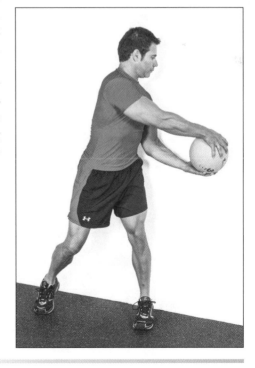

CHAPTER 6

LEGS AND HIPS

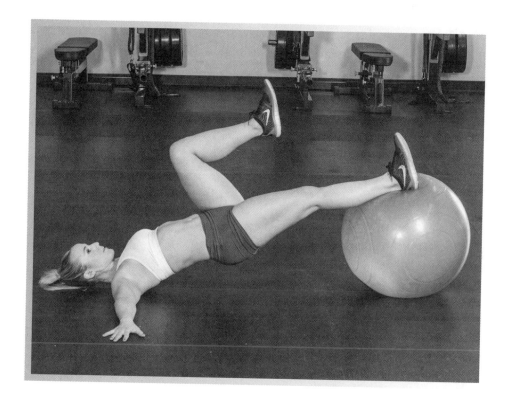

Hip Extension and Knee Flexion

This is the only exercise that can work your hamstrings as both a knee flexor and hip extensor, making this an extremely functional and productive exercise.

Setup

Lying supine on the floor, place a ball under your heels. Arms are in a T position to assist in balance.

Movement

Initiate movement by squeezing your glutes and raising your hips off the floor. Once you reach the position in which your ankles, knees, and hips are in line, bring your heels toward you by flexing your knees.

Finish

Once your heels have gone to their end range, reverse the movement. Extend the knees, then lower your hips.

Tips and Progressions

- Move your arms in from a T position to your sides.
- Use a larger ball to increase your range of motion and improve balance.
- Add a cable or surgical tubing around your ankle to increase the load as your knees flex.
- Use a single-leg movement instead of a double-leg movement.

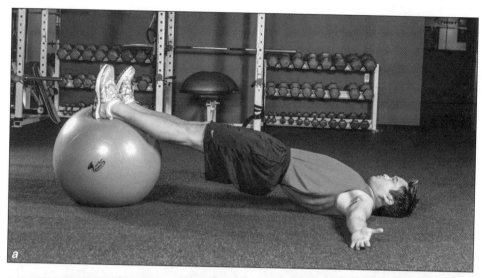

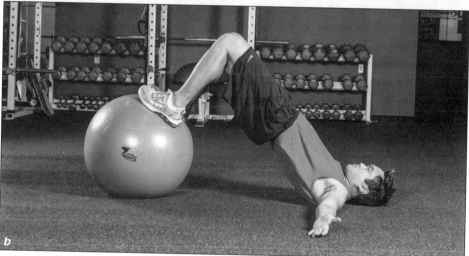

Knee Tuck

This exercise targets the lower abdominals and hip flexors by having you lift a loaded ball.

Setup

Lie flat on the floor, supine. Back is flat, core is set, and legs are extended. Hold a DSL stability ball between the feet. Rest your arms alongside your torso.

Movement

Keep your back and hips on the floor as you flex the knees to draw the feet toward your body. Tuck the knees in tight over your torso; pause.

Finish

Extend the legs under control, allowing the heels to touch the floor at the extreme range.

Tips and Progressions

- Initially it may be necessary to place your arms out to the sides for stability or to press the arms into the floor during the lift phase. Eventually your goal is to keep your arms relaxed during the lower-body lift.
- If you note excessive lumbar arch or back discomfort, try wedging your hands underneath the glutes.
- If the loaded ball is too heavy, you lose your anchored position, or you still experience low back discomfort, regress to an unweighted ABS ball and complete supplemental ball bridge exercises.

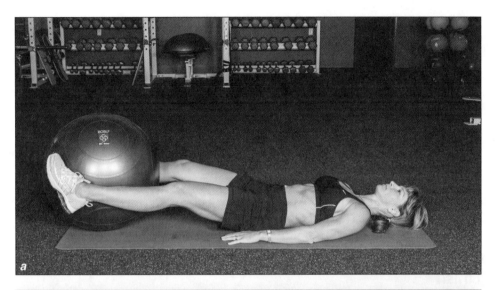

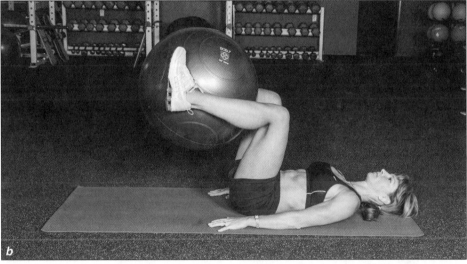

Poor Man's Glute Ham Raise Rollout

This is called a poor man's exercise because there is no expensive glute ham raise bench involved in performing this exercise. It is an excellent movement that focuses on the hamstrings, glutes, and low back.

Setup

Kneel in front of a ball and perform a pelvic tilt, moving your glutes forward and drawing in your navel toward your spine. Place your hands on top of the ball, and have a partner hold your ankles down. As with the kneeling rollout, instead of your core doing the work, the focus is on your hamstrings and posterior chain.

Movement

Your hands remain stationary on the ball. Pivot on your knees, and bring your torso and hips forward as the ball rolls away from your knees. Contract your hamstrings by applying pressure upward on your partner's hands with your ankles. This results in eccentric lengthening of your hamstrings.

Finish

Once you have loaded yourself eccentrically, contract your hamstrings and pull yourself back up to the starting position. Do not release the pressure you exert into your partner's hands.

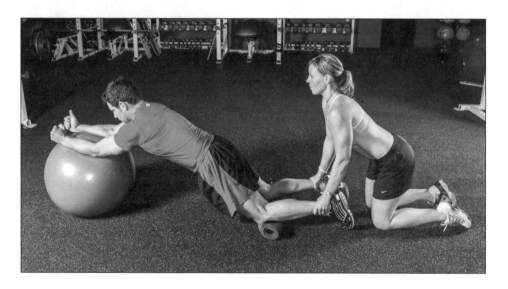

Lateral Wall Squat

The lateral wall squat builds sport-specific strength, replicating the angles needed for lateral movement and stopping. The glutes, hamstrings, and quadriceps are the main targets of this exercise.

Setup

Stand sideways beside a wall. Position a stability ball against the wall at elbow height. Lean against the ball at a 45-degree angle, your outside leg supporting your body weight.

Movement

Lower into a one-leg squat position, maintaining the 45-degree angle and leaning into the ball. As you flex your knee and lower your hips, the ball will move from elbow height to shoulder height. Keep your hips and shoulders as square as possible.

Finish

Using the muscles in your support leg, extend the leg to elevate your body back to the setup position.

Tips and Progressions

To increase the difficulty of the exercise, repeat the exercise using your inside leg.

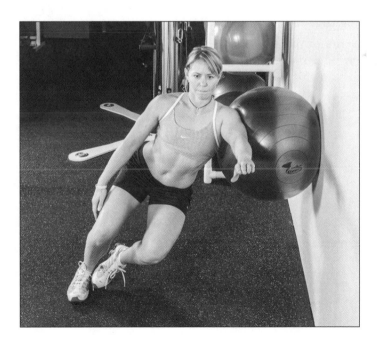

Alternating Stability Ball Hip Extension With Single-Leg Eccentric Knee Flexion

Research has proven the importance of eccentric work for the hamstrings in helping protect and support the knee ligaments and the integrity of the entire knee. This integrated movement focuses on eccentric loading.

Setup

Place your feet on top of a strength ball with your body lying on the floor and arms placed in a T position or by your sides.

Movement

Squeeze your glutes and engage your core and lift your hips off the floor. Keep your hips up and pull the ball toward you with your heels as you would in the hip extension knee flexion exercise.

Finish

Remove one foot from the ball and extend your leg back out on its own. Once you are fully extended, place your foot back on the ball so both feet are on top and repeat the same motion on the other side. The loading of the single leg should take 4 to 5 seconds in a slow movement.

Tips and Progressions

- Keeping your core engaged and your hips up is key to this movement.
- If you cannot maintain your positioning as you transition to a single-leg support or cannot move in the recommended 4 to 5 seconds, you may not be ready for this exercise.

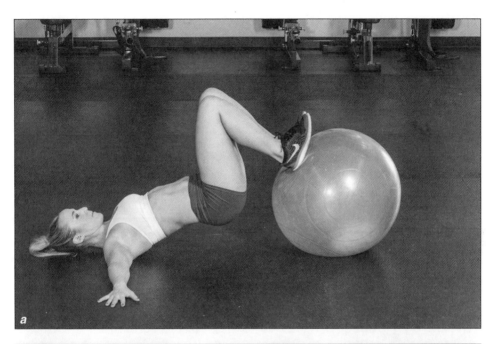

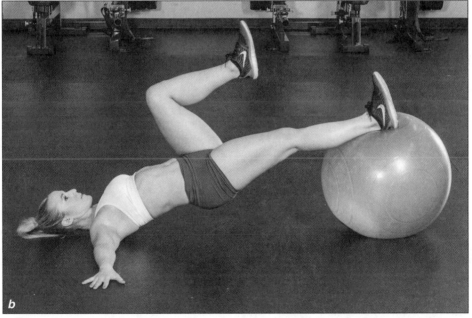

Stability Ball Split Squat With Dumbbell

This movement focuses on leg strength and core stability.

Setup

Stand with your back against a stability ball pressed into a wall. Assume a split position so that your front leg is at a 90-degree angle. Hold a dumbbell in the hand opposite the front leg with your arm in a down position. Using only one dumbbell will engage your core to one side as you attempt to hold a neutral spine in the frontal plane.

Movement

Move up and down in a split squat position, allowing the ball to roll behind you on the wall. Move in a controlled manner while maintaining your core, not allowing your body to shift at all. Lower your knee to come within 1 inch (2.5 cm) of the floor.

Finish

Ensure you are completing full reps by extending your hip at the top position.

Tips and Progressions

Control your movement. Do not use momentum to propel yourself out of the bottom position.

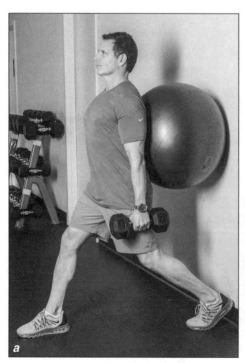
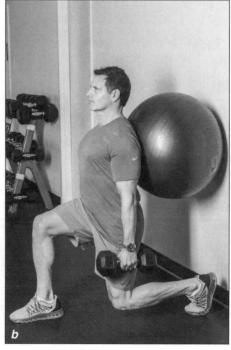

Repeated Dual-Foot Long Jump

Similar to the box jump, this exercise focuses more on horizontal power.

Setup

Stand with feet hip-width apart holding a medicine ball at chest height close to your body.

Movement

Rapidly dropping your hips, explode forward in a horizontal fashion, whereby you attempt to drive your hips into extension as you rise off the floor. Drive the medicine ball into the air forward, enhancing full body extension.

Finish

After you have come off the floor, land with a tall body but with soft hips, knees, and ankles to absorb the landing, and finish in a tall position.

Tips and Progressions

- Do not land with fully flexed hips.
- Reset before each jump.

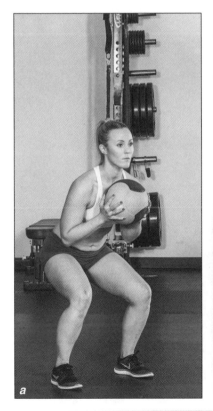
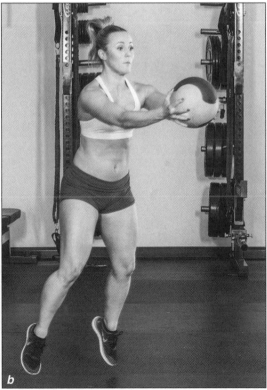

Stability Ball Side-Supported Hip Extension

This movement is great for those seeking to focus on the hip abductors and hip adductors.

Setup

Set up laterally on a stability ball, with the ball placed on your side and your arm draped around the ball. Feet are on the floor stacked on top of each other and acting as a support for your lower body. Focus on the adductors similar as described but your top leg is flexed and planted directly on the floor.

Movement

To focus on the abductors, raise your leg off of the other one and hold for a second(*a*). To focus on the adductors(*b*), raise the lower leg as high as you can and hold this position.

Finish

Bring each leg to the start position before completing the next rep. Complete all the abductor movements first and switch to the adductor movements.

Tips and Progressions

By adding an ankle weight, you can increase the intensity of this movement.

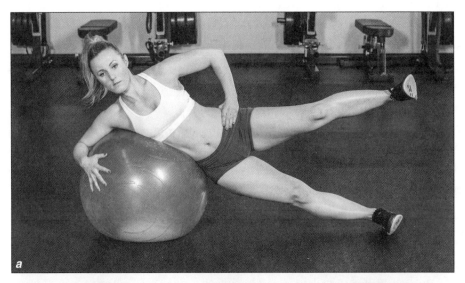

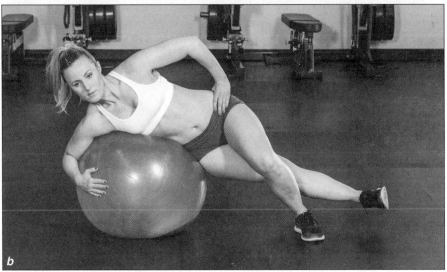

Plyometric Medicine Ball Box Jump

Box jumps have become very prevalent in the fitness industry. Any type of jump can be considered high-intensity loading, and you must take care regarding technique.

Setup

Stand in front of a knee-high box holding a medicine ball at chest height close to your body.

Movement

Rapidly dropping your hips, you will want to explode up in a vertical fashion, whereby you attempt to drive your hips into extension as you rise off the floor. The medicine ball should be driven into the air, enhancing full body extension.

Finish

After you have come off the floor, you will land with a tall body but with soft hips, knees, and ankles to absorb the landing and finish in a tall position.

Tips and Progressions

- Do not land with fully flexed hips.
- Do not jump down to begin your next rep. Step down with control and reset.

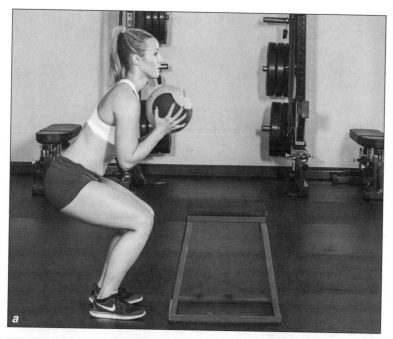

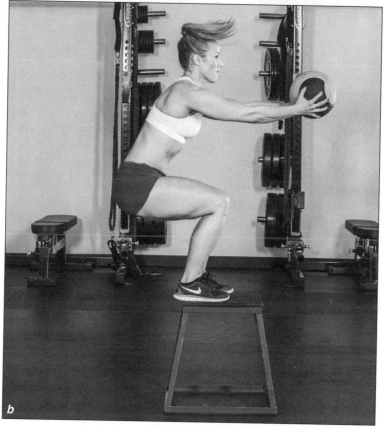

Single-Leg Stride Squat

The core control and glute strength to express both the single-leg squat and stride patterns are relevant abilities for most human motion.

Setup

Hold a medicine ball in both hands in an athletic-ready position: quads loaded, hips dropped, torso upright.

Movement

Pick up one foot, extending the leg back at a 45-degree angle to stride out behind the body. The loaded leg lowers into a deep squat. Press the medicine ball diagonally away from the extended foot to the opposite side of the body.

Finish

Get length (through full body between medicine ball and back foot) and pause; hold without touching the back foot down. This is very challenging. Be sure to fully extend (straighten) the back leg. When achieved, the glutes will noticeably scream.

Tips and Progressions

- Squatting, striding, and pushing at the same time are an incredible challenge of the entire body. Very common mechanical breakdowns are a triple play—coming up tall on the squat leg, falling into forward torso flexion, and holding a bent back leg. Together these three errors eliminate the potential exercise benefits.
- Progress this exercise by lowering deeper into the squat, striding fully by holding the heel of the foot higher while retaining a taller torso; reach to full arm extension.
- Adding pauses in the most challenging position is an incredible demand in advancing strength. Time pauses, progressing the duration over a set number of workouts.

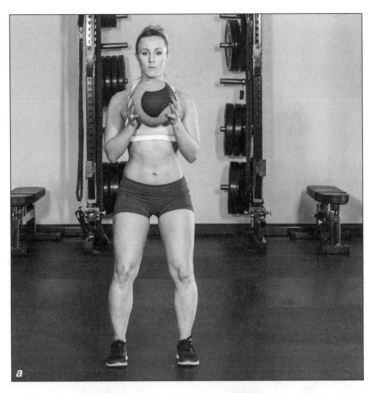

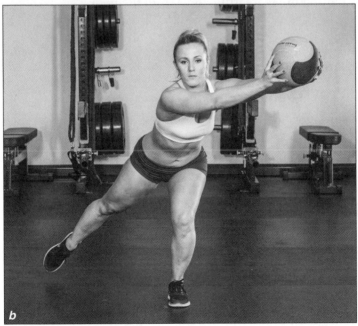

Wall Squat

The squat is a foundational strength exercise from which many other leg exercises build. Wall squats are technically easier to execute and allow those with low back problems to participate. This exercise encourages a deeper range of motion and static holds at the bottom while retaining a solid postural position.

Setup

Begin facing away from the wall. Place a stability ball between the wall and your back, positioned level with the lumbar vertebrae. Lean your weight against the ball and adjust your feet, shuffling them out away from your body. Ensure a shoulder-width stance with the feet forward and toes pointed slightly outward.

Movement

To initiate movement, press the heels into the floor to engage the deep abdominal wall. Set the core before slowly lowering your hips toward the floor, flexing the knees until the tibias are perpendicular to the floor with a 90-degree angle at the knees.

Middle Position

In the middle position you should feel a strong load in the quads and glutes while the knees are working but comfortable. Eyes look straight forward, and neck is in a neutral position. If you sense too much strain on the knees, visually check to ensure your knees are not out past your toes. If they are, readjust your setup position by moving the feet farther away from the body.

Finish

Extend the legs to push the body back up the wall to a standing position. Retain pressure against the ball during the entire range of motion.

Tips and Progressions

- Use a slow movement tempo, counting 2 seconds on the concentric and eccentric phases.
- To advance the challenge, integrate a static hold at the middle position for each repetition, holding that deep stance for 3 to 5 seconds before rising back up.
- To emphasize the core, lift one foot 2 centimeters (less than 1 inch) off the floor during each static hold, focusing on retaining a level pelvis.
- To increase the strength demands, hold dumbbells at your sides with arms slightly flexed and palms facing in toward the body.

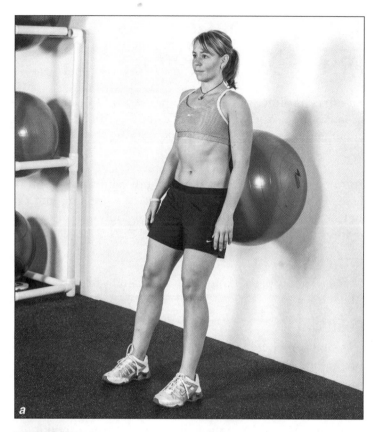

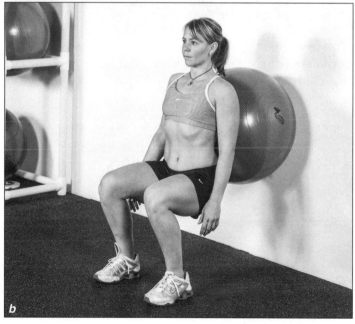

O'Brien Hip Extension
With Static Hip Flexion

The O'Brien hip extension was shown to me by Andy O'Brien, a strength coach for the Florida Panthers, during a training camp. It is an excellent exercise that focuses on maintaining pelvic position while working the glutes.

Setup

Begin in a prone position over the ball with both hands placed on the floor to provide a base. The right leg is flexed with the knee pressing into the ball with approximately 30 percent effort. This static hip flexion will offset the hip extension on the opposite side to maintain a solid pelvis.

Movement

Once your knee is solidly placed into the ball, begin by firing your left glute and extending the left leg.

Middle Position

The left leg should be extended to a point at which the knee, hip, and shoulder create a straight line. Hold this position for 2 to 3 seconds.

Finish

After holding the middle position, slowly lower the leg to the start position without releasing the right flexed hip into the ball. Complete your repetitions on the left leg, then reverse the position for the right leg.

Tips and Progressions

If you feel tension or pain in your lower back, this may be a result of weak gluteal muscles. You should check with a therapist or doctor for direction if you have pain.

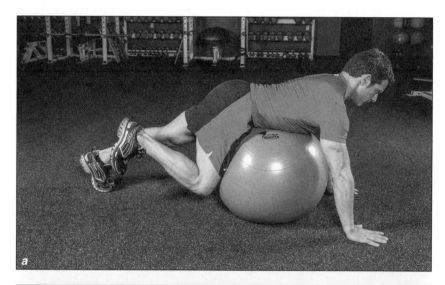

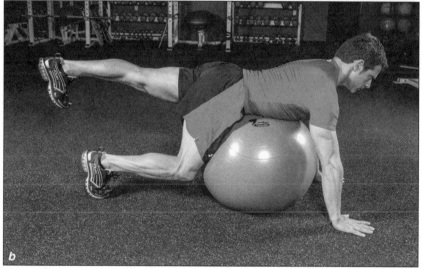

Single-Leg Squat

Training one leg at a time transfers strength gains to the sport environment, where movement is achieved one leg at a time. Incorporating the stability ball facilitates a deeper range of motion and also assists in the concentric positive phase back to a standing position. A DSL ball will stay in place so you can drop your glutes onto it.

Setup

Begin in a seated position, hips on the top front side of the DSL stability ball, centering one foot on the floor at the midline of your body. Sit up tall and set the core. The opposite foot is extended forward.

Movement

Lift up and extend the grounded leg to a standing position. Balance before returning, under control, to a seated position.

Tips and Progressions

- Use a controlled bounce to help initiate the concentric lift phase if you are unable to rise up to stand from a static seated position.
- Always double-check that the DSL stability ball is perfectly in place behind you for each rep.
- If one leg is not as strong, begin your first set with that leg and finish your last set with that leg—effectively completing one extra set for the weaker leg.

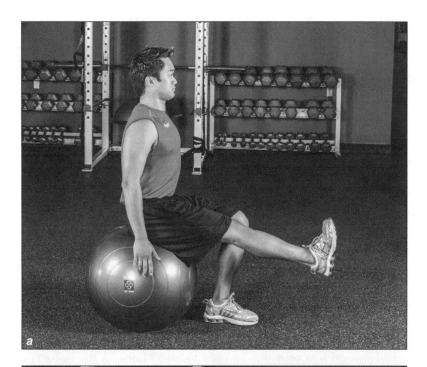

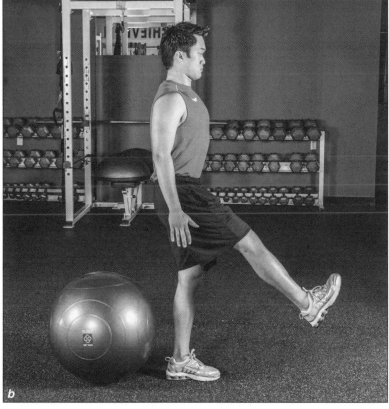

Goldy's Leg Blaster

The inner and outer thighs are two areas that athletes have always had a difficult time training. Most exercises for these areas are completed with the foot off the floor (with the multihip machine or cable attachments). The problem with these exercises is that they don't transfer to actual sport situations. The inner and outer thigh muscles are most often used in movements that require the foot to be in contact with the floor. The leg blaster can train these muscles in this manner.

Setup

Set up close to an adjustable-cable column using a 45-centimeter ball. Place a cable belt around your inside ankle, with your foot sitting on top of the ball. The outside leg is your plant and should maintain a bent-knee position. Your hips are back, and your abdominals are set. This setup method emphasizes the inner thighs and quads.

Movement

To activate the inner-thigh muscles, the initial movement comes from the inside of the foot pressing down on the ball. Once you have established this pressure, roll the ball toward you by bringing your hip in. Maintain the natural curve in your lower back and keep the hips back.

Finish

Return to the starting position by releasing your leg, allowing it a full range of motion on the return.

Tips and Variations

You can also focus on the outer-thigh muscles by placing the cable on the opposite leg, as described previously. The movement and sequence are the same, but the main difference is that you push out instead of pull in.

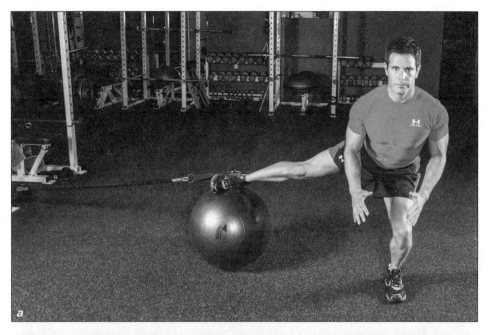

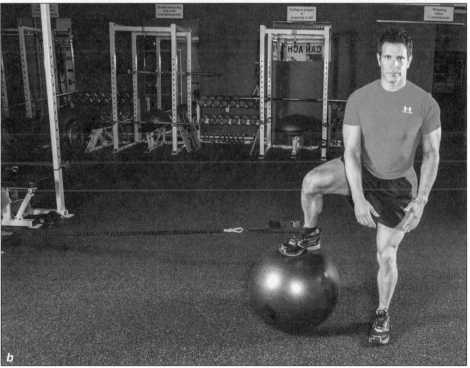

Hip Power Initiation

Most athletes have imbalances in hip mobility caused by body structure (such as a difference in leg lengths) and repetitive actions specific to the mechanics of their sports. This exercise exposes imbalances while strengthening two key movements: inward and outward rotation. A goal is to isolate the hips from the trunk; you aim to keep the chest facing the floor and the shoulders square while the hips rotate. While the goal is to minimize trunk rotation, the hip power achieved through this exercise contributes to rotary power either from the top down (as in swinging a tennis racket) or from the ground up (as in pivoting to change direction).

Setup

Begin crouched behind the stability ball. Move on top of the ball and walk out with the hands until you are in a short-lever push-up position with the knees on the ball. Flex the knees to bring the feet up in the air. Hold the legs and feet together. Select a ball size that allows a level line from knee to shoulder.

Movement

Keeping the trunk and shoulders square to the floor, rotate at the hips—think of two pivot points, one on each side of the hips. Rotate the hips to place the ball and knees out to the side of the body. Return through to the opposite side of the body, alternating sides.

Tips and Progressions

- Begin with a slow tempo to safely build strength, stability, control, and range of motion.
- Once you've achieved all these and have them well trained over several workouts, you can vary the tempo, with a goal of fast movement. Rotate to the left and immediately reverse direction to the opposite side, where you pause at each rep. This focuses power initiation off one side. The eccentric–concentric coupling builds power initiation.
- You can also move at a higher pace with fluidity from side to side without pausing.

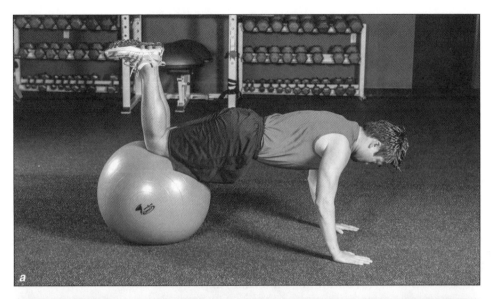

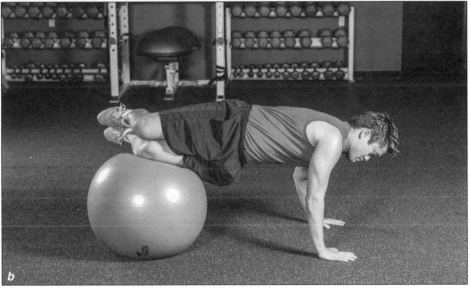

Prone Ball Hold With Knee Drive

This exercise helps you build premovement core activation and trunk stability to hold a push-up position and stabilize yourself on the ball. It also works the lower abdominals and hip flexors when you add leg movement. Holding your body weight on the ball preloads the core for stabilization and movement. The best way to understand this is to experience it.

Setup

Assume a push-up position with the heels of the hands on the upper out-side of the ball and fingers wrapped down the ball. Feet are on the floor, up on toes in a shoulder-width stance. With straight arms, sink into the middle back before flexing the elbows two inches (5 cm). Load your body weight onto the arms and engage the core.

Movement

Slowly bring the knee of one leg straight up as close to the chest as possible, pause, and return. Switch legs, bringing the knee of the opposite leg in toward the chest, pause, and continue to alternate legs.

Middle Position

Progress by lengthening the pause in the middle position for each rep. If the longer hold results in a rounded back, return to regular fluid reps with no pause.

Tips and Progressions

- For an advanced progression that increases activation of the transverse abdominis and internal hip rotators, pull the knee in and over to the opposite elbow. Begin with a slow, controlled tempo along with a half-second pause at the middle position.
- To progress, first lengthen the pauses.
- Once you have built the strength to handle this, increase the speed of movement, driving the knee to the opposite elbow before holding.

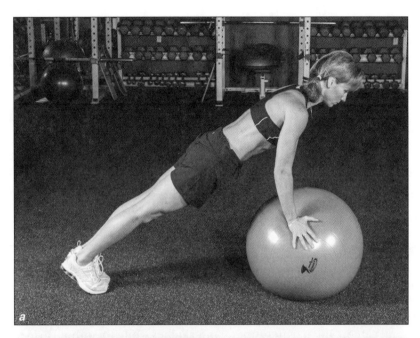

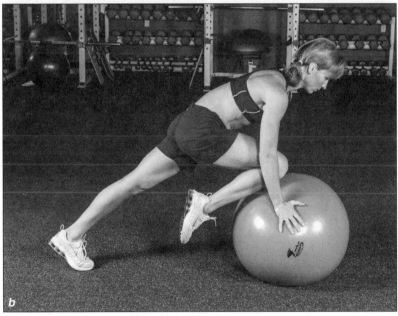

Lunge With Medicine Ball Pass

This complex exercise takes an important leg strength exercise and adds upper-body power.

Setup

Partners face each other, about three to four strides apart. One partner has a medicine ball.

Movement

While holding the ball, lift one leg off the floor, flexing at the hip and knee, and cycle it forward to softly plant it on the floor ahead of the body. The lunge length is long enough to produce a 90-degree angle at the knee (your knee cannot go past your toes) and low enough that your thigh is parallel to the floor. Before landing, pass the ball toward your partner.

Finish

Hold the lunge position and focus to remain well balanced. While receiving the return pass, push off with your lead foot to return to the starting position.

Tips and Progressions

Lunge and catch: One partner lunges and catches while the other throws. Alternate lunging with the left and right leg while receiving passes at random. Your partner passes directly in front of you to a variety of places outside your midline and changes position to deliver passes across your body (passes sent from off to the side). The pass reception sequence is always catch, balance, and hold for 2 seconds before returning the ball to your partner and taking your next lunge step.

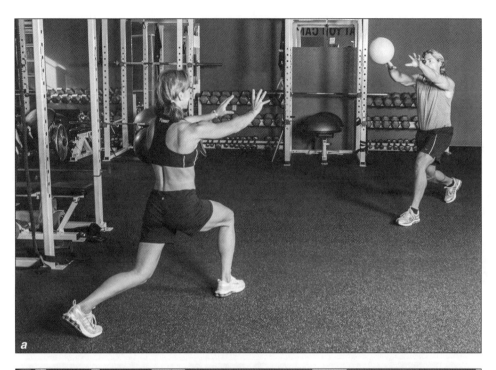

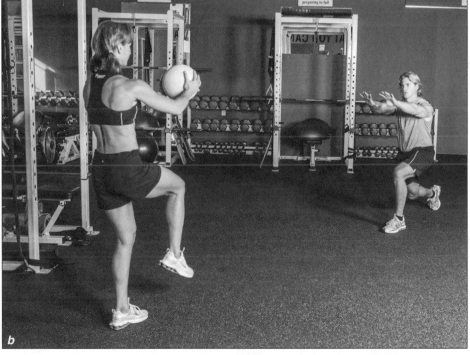

Reverse Lunge and Rotate

This exercise encourages thoracic spine freedom of motion through the transverse plane and extends range of motion throughout the legs and hips.

Setup

Stand in an athletic-ready position, holding a medicine ball in front of the torso.

Movement

Pick up one foot, reaching back to plant the foot directly behind the body and landing as far back as possible. Keeping the torso upright and body balanced, slowly rotate around across the front support leg.

Finish

Reverse the rotary action back to neutral before kicking off the back foot, rising up to athletic-ready setup stance.

Tips and Progressions

Focus on reaching with the rear foot to finish longer and deeper into that reverse lunge and sustain a taller torso.

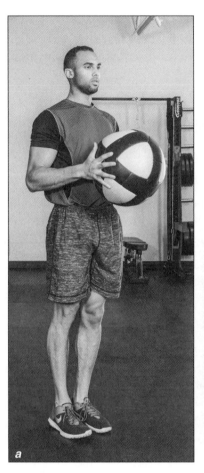 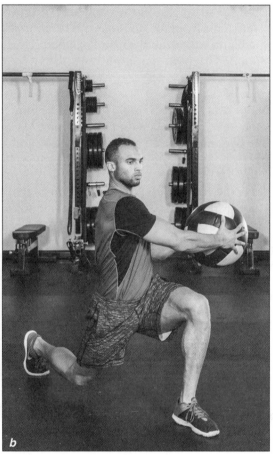

Lunge to Press and Track

Develop stride strength, challenge single-leg balance, and improve muscle sequencing from toes to fingertips for more functional muscle recruitment when you blend legs, shoulders, and balance. The heavier the medicine ball, the more shoulder strength required.

Setup

Stand balanced on a single leg while holding a medicine ball in one hand at the shoulder on the same side as the support leg. Set and brace the core, and establish a strong middle back. Steady the ankle, and slightly flex the knee.

Movement

Cycle the free leg up and out in front of the body in as long a stride as possible. Land softly—heel first—rolling to the full foot as you shift your weight forward, keeping the medicine ball at the shoulder. Keeping the head up, chest lifted, and abdominal muscles tight, slowly lower your hips toward the floor until the back knee is just above the floor and the lead knee is flexed to about 90 degrees with the upper leg parallel to the floor. If the front knee is ahead of that foot, spread the feet farther apart.

Middle Position

Shift body weight forward to the lead foot, and forcefully push off the floor by extending the front hip and knee. Let the effort come from the front leg to achieve a standing position as you press the medicine ball overhead. The back knee drives forward, finishing at waist height. From this single-leg balanced position with the arm remaining fully extended, lower the medicine ball laterally until the arm is parallel to the floor, pause slightly, then raise the medicine ball back up overhead. Pass it across to complete the same movements with the opposite arm.

Finish

Pass the ball back to your original arm, lower the medicine ball back to the shoulder, reach and step back into the lunge position, and drive off the lead leg back into a single-leg standing position.

Tips and Progressions

- To advance the challenge, visually track the medicine ball to the side. Begin tracking with just your eyes. Think of tunnel vision, where your eyes watch only the medicine ball.
- Advance to moving your entire head to follow the ball. Tilt your head to look up at the ball.
- You can also increase the weight of the medicine ball.

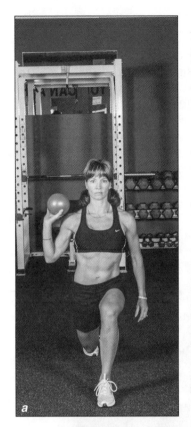

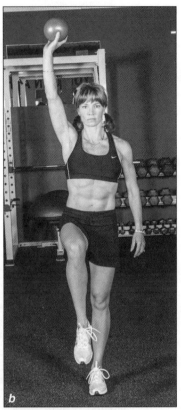

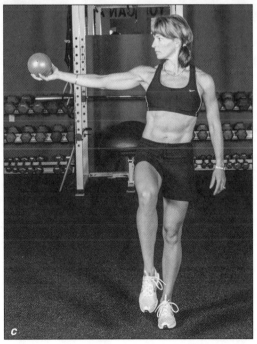

Single-Leg Rotations

Most athletes have imbalances in hip mobility caused by body structure (such as a difference in leg lengths) and repetitive actions specific to the mechanics of their sports. This exercise exposes imbalances while strengthening two key movements: inward and outward rotation. A goal is to isolate the hips from the trunk; you aim to keep the chest facing the floor and the shoulders square while the hips rotate. The improved hip strength contributes to rotary power, lateral deceleration, and stride movement patterns.

Setup

Begin crouched behind the stability ball. Move on top of the ball and walk out with your hands until you are in a prone push-up position with feet on the ball. Release one foot.

Movement

Move the knee of the free leg down and around the body as the leg on the ball rotates to the inside. Unwind this movement and continue past neutral (setup) position, moving the free leg up and over the body. The goal is to touch the foot to the floor on the opposite side of the body.

Finish

Return back to the prone setup position. Adjust the foot on the ball if necessary before entering the next repetition.

Tips and Progressions

- This exercise looks complex, but it is very achievable. In the learning stage, it is easy for the leg to fall off the ball during rotation. Practice with a spotter behind the ball whose hands will "bookend" the ball, allowing the ball to travel only an inch (~2.5 cm) in either direction.

- In your workout, make sure this exercise does not follow a tough chest-push set; otherwise it will be difficult to hold the setup position for the desired rep count.

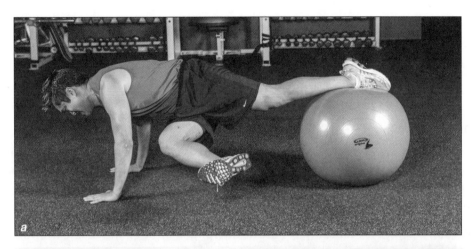

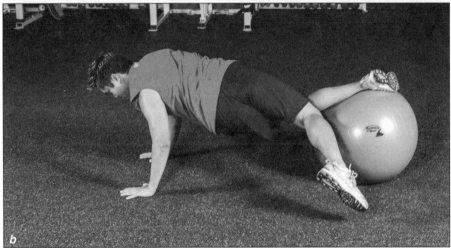

Kneeling Side Pass

This exercise works the hips and torso with a frontal plane loading through side flexion of the trunk.

Setup

Partners stand 4 feet (1.2 m) apart, both facing the same wall. One partner has a medicine ball. Begin in a kneeling position with the torso upright.

Movement

Partner A passes to partner B. Partner B catches the ball above head height, about an inch (2.5 cm) in front of the body. Absorb the catch and follow through as far as possible to the opposite side while keeping the torso upright.

Finish

Partner B brings the ball back overhead and follows through with a side-overhead pass back to partner A.

Tips and Progressions

Standing catch: Position the feet shoulder-width apart. Flex the knees and set the abdominals. Turn the head to see your partner. Catch the ball above head height and about an inch in front of your body, but follow through farther to the opposite side. If accuracy allows, move farther apart to require more power on the throw and more load on the catch reception.

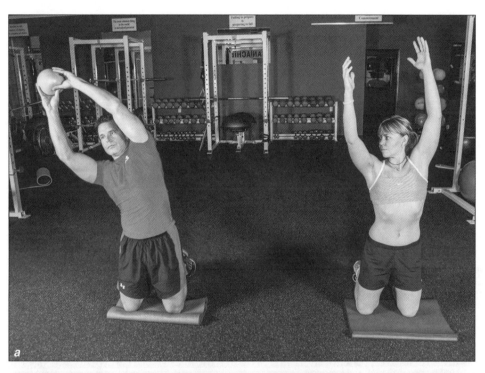

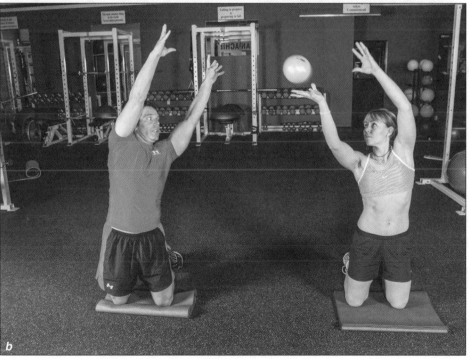

Lateral Squat With Ball Push

This is a great full-body exercise. You will feel this in the legs, back, core, and shoulders.

Setup

Stand with feet at shoulder width. Hold a medicine ball with two hands in front of the body.

Movement

Step out to the left and lower into a lateral squat position, shifting body weight over the left leg. As you lower over the left leg, push the medicine ball out away from your chest until arms are fully extended. Hold this position for 2 seconds.

Finish

Push off the left leg to move back into a neutral stance. As you push off the left leg, pull the ball back in toward your chest. Next, step out to the right, and extend your arms to push the ball out away from your chest and lower into a side squat position. Hold for 2 seconds. Push off the right leg and pull the ball back in to return to the start position.

Tips and Progressions

As an alternative you can alternate pressing the ball overhead with each lateral lunge changing the resultant forces of gravity as a result of the position.

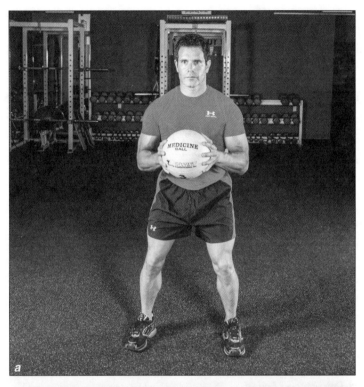

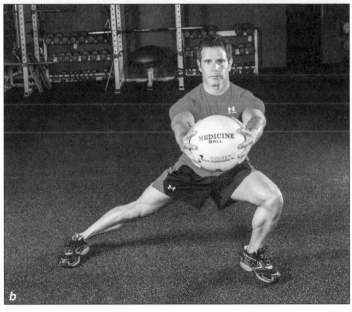

Squat Press

This exercise combines a squat and sit-up with arms fully extended under load. Use a DSL stability ball to safely execute the movement pattern while holding dumbbells.

Setup

Set your DSL stability ball in neutral ball position (label up). The DSL stability ball has circle markings that can be used as a reference point in an effort to complete the supine portion without ball movement and to define a target spot to aim for that will help you avoid falling off the ball.

Begin in a standing position in front of the DSL stability ball. Feet are shoulder-width apart, core is set and braced, and middle back is set. Hold light dumbbells above your head (in a shoulder press position), arms extended.

Movement

Maintaining solid posture, squat by lowering the hips into a seated position so that the glutes touch at about the outer edge of the large top circle. Sit down on the top front side of your DSL stability ball, keeping the arms extended overhead. Lie back into a bridge position, arms still extended, now up over the chest.

Finish

Sit up off the DSL ball, shifting the arms overhead so that you stand up with arms extended overhead.

Tips and Progressions

- Learn this exercise with no dumbbells but assume the same arm position.
- Next, begin with the lightest weight and progress step by step. The load you can handle will be limited by strength, stability, and flexibility in the shoulders and back.

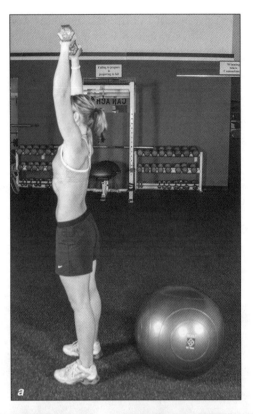

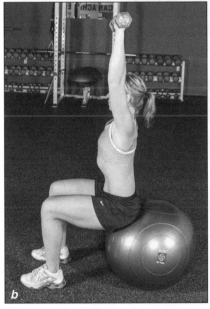

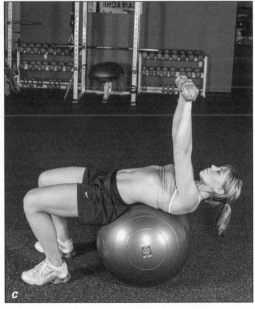

Leg–Hip–Core Multidirectional Control

The purpose of this exercise is not to apply the greatest force, such as during a leg press. It challenges the inner unit to stabilize the supine position while the hips and legs adjust position.

Setup

Lie on the floor with your knees flexed. You and your partner together hold a stability ball between your feet. Increase the foot pressure on the ball to lift it up until the lower legs are parallel to the floor.

Movement

Cooperatively move the ball forward, backward, up, down, and sideways while keeping the back flat on the floor.

Tips and Progressions

Complete the same exercise with each partner using only one leg, as shown in the photo.

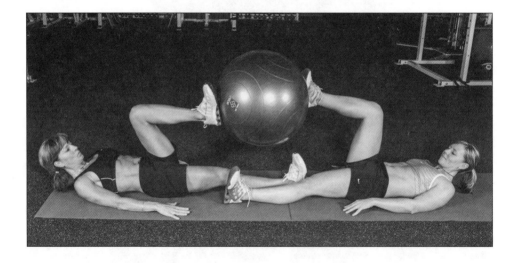

CHAPTER 7

CHEST

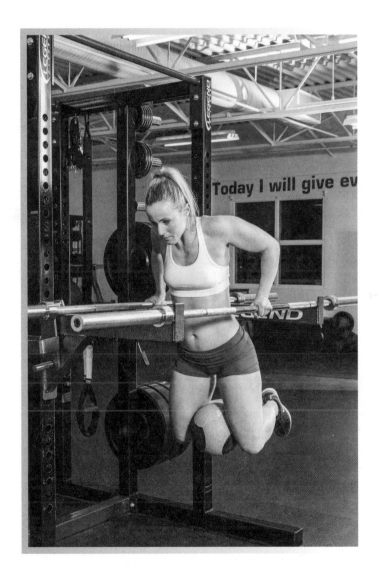

Incline Dumbbell Press

The incline dumbbell press focuses on the upper pectoral muscles. This exercise is typically performed on an incline bench, but you can perform it on a ball to incorporate the elements of balance and stability to the upper extremity.

Setup

A larger ball is necessary for the correct support. Holding dumbbells, sit on a ball, and slowly walk out to a position in which your head, shoulders, and back are supported by the ball. Ensure that your feet are slightly wider than hip width to provide a safe initial base of support.

Movement

Begin by setting your abdominals and pressing your arms in an upward arc to the point where your hands are over your eyes.

Finish

Once you have reached the top position, return the dumbbells to a point where they touch the tops of your shoulders.

Tips and Progressions

You can increase the difficulty of this exercise by using the following methods:

- Decrease the width of your feet to increase the stability factor for this exercise.
- Perform a one-arm dumbbell press to greatly increase the difficulty of this exercise; this will require greater core stabilization.

Safety Notes

- Ensure that the floor is clean and dust free. As you press into the ball on an angle, a clean and dust-free floor will help in preventing the ball from rolling out and away from you.
- The hand position shown is the traditional grip. A neutral grip, in which the palms face each other, places the shoulders under less stress than the traditional bench press position. In the traditional position the palms face away and the shoulders are externally rotated. If you have any kind of shoulder ailment, you should use the neutral grip position.

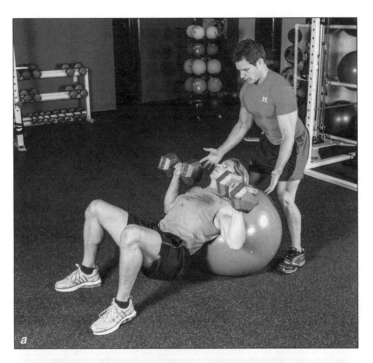

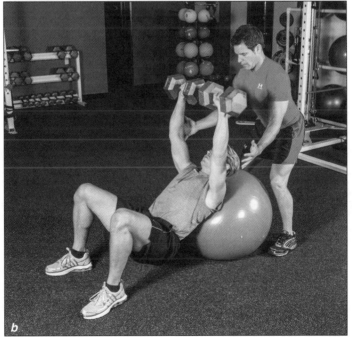

Supine Push and Drive

This exercise takes the old dumbbell bench press and turns it into something much more functional for shoulder and core development. Although this has been designated as a chest exercise, significant core rotation is demonstrated here.

Setup

Begin by holding a single dumbbell in your right hand and sitting on a stability ball. Walk out so that you are in the tabletop position with your head and shoulders supported by the ball. Activate your core and especially your glutes. The right arm is set in the bottom position of a dumbbell press.

Movement

From the bottom position, drive the dumbbell up and toward the midline of the body, as you would in a standard dumbbell bench press.

Finish

Just as you are about to reach full extension of your arm, rotate your body and continue to drive the weight. The momentum will cause you to roll to your left, and you will end up being supported by your left arm.

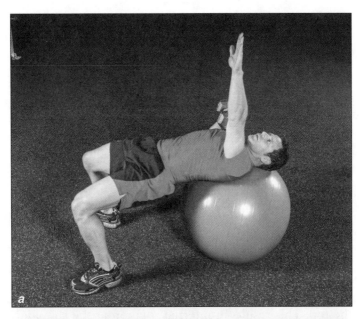

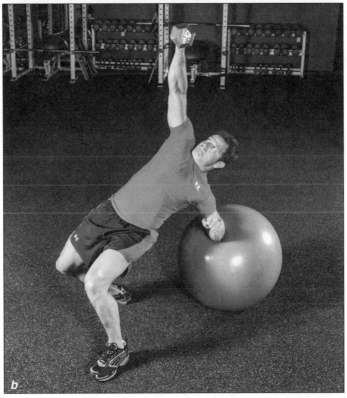

Supine Dumbbell Press and Fly

This exercise provides a great challenge to the pectorals because it combines two popular movements for the chest. The supine dumbbell press and fly also requires great coordination.

Setup

With dumbbells in each hand, sit on a stability ball and roll out so you are in a tabletop position. One arm is in a flexed position, or the bottom position of a dumbbell bench press. The other arm is in a position similar to the bottom position of a dumbbell fly with a slight bend in the elbow. Glutes and core are activated to provide a stable base for movement.

Movement

The concentric movement begins with the bench press arm and the fly arm initiating movement at the same time. The fly-arm angle at the elbow should not change during the lifting.

Finish

Both dumbbells meet over the top of the chest. The press-side arm supinates as you reach the top. This results in internal rotation at the shoulder, which will assist in a more effective contraction of the pectoralis major. Complete your set on one side and then switch arm positions.

Tips and Progressions

- By changing your hand position on the dumbbells, you can target different parts of your pectoral muscle. Try varying your grip from prone to supine to neutral.
- You can add a weight vest or sandbag over your abdominals to increase the activity of the core and glutes.

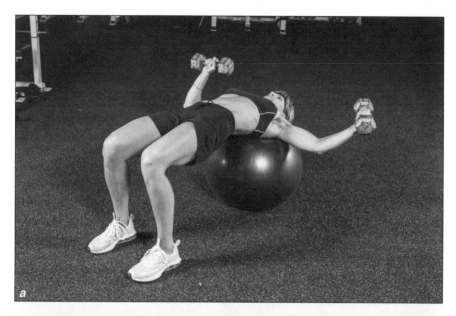

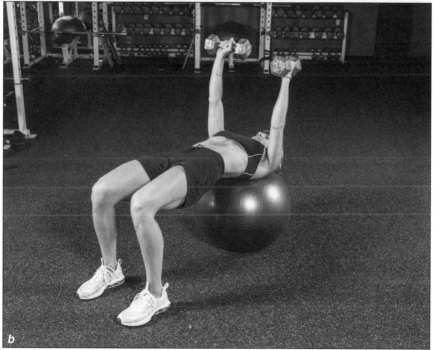

Dual-Ball Fly

This is the perfect replacement for the pec deck. Not only do you work your chest in a very demanding exercise, but you also work your entire body as you attempt to maintain proper posture.

Setup

Bring two stability balls together, side by side. Place each of your lower arms on a ball. Your body is on a 45-degree angle, with normal curvature of your low back.

Movement

Begin movement by rolling the balls outward and allowing your arms to open up. Move to a point where you feel you have reached a comfortable range of motion. If you have any kind of shoulder problem, you should avoid this exercise because it places great stress on the anterior capsule of the shoulder.

Finish

Once you have reached the range of motion that you are comfortable with, squeeze your arms back together, bringing the balls back to the start position.

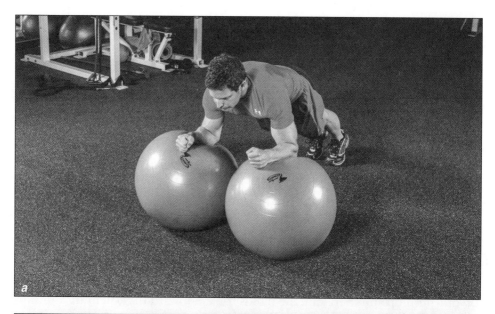

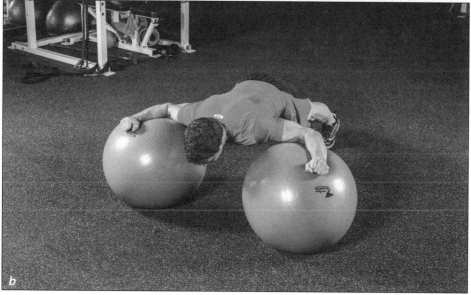

Walk-Out to Push-Up

This exercise challenges the upper-body musculature while requiring core strength and stabilization. This is an excellent shoulder stabilization exercise that works the posterior deltoids.

Setup

Standing behind the ball, crouch down and place your abdominals on top of the ball. Roll forward until your hands reach the floor in front of the ball. Walk your hands out until your hips are off the ball and your quadriceps rest on top of the ball.

Movement

Focus on maintaining a strong core by contracting the postural muscles to keep the hips up strong and the body aligned. (Prevent hips from sagging, and avoid any hip or torso rotation.) Walk your hands out until your feet remain on top of the ball.

Finish

Do one push-up and then walk the hands back in toward the ball until your hips are once again on top of the ball. Pay close attention to the movement of your shoulder blades. If you have a winging or protruding shoulder blade as you lower yourself, you should avoid this exercise and seek medical advice.

Tips and Progressions

- When you complete the push-up, hold only one foot on top of the ball. The other leg is removed at the far position of each rep and held straight.
- Walk out as fast as you can, then to return back to the ball, jump with both hands together in a plyometric action, and shuffle back to the setup position.
- Walk out as slowly as you can, supporting yourself on only one hand for an extended time. Keep your hips up strong and aligned without hip or torso rotation; your shoulders and hips should face square to the floor.

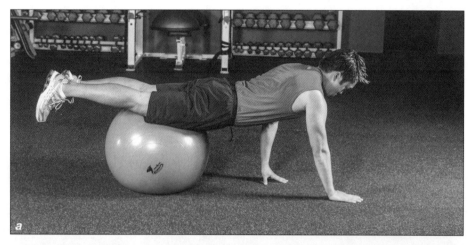

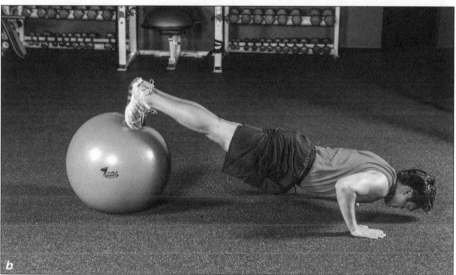

Jump-Out to Push-Up

This is a dynamic upper-body plyometric exercise for training power. Most people are used to the feeling of jumping in the legs. The same abilities are needed in the upper body to fuel sport skills and avoid injury when absorbing falls. It uses a deceleration–acceleration coupling through the eccentric (landing and braking) and concentric (jumping) phases. You should be competent in doing push-ups and also capable of completing sets of walk-out push-ups before progressing to this exercise.

Setup

Begin crouched behind the stability ball. Roll onto the ball, extend the arms in front of the body, and set the core and middle back.

Movement

Roll right over the ball until the hands reach the floor. Absorb the landing and immediately extend the arms with enough power to release the hands from the floor.

Aim each subsequent landing a little farther away from the ball, carrying the body out to a full push-up position with the feet on the ball. Jump with the hands back in toward the ball all the way to the crouched setup position.

Tips and Progressions

- When first trying this exercise, try to land softly and move through each partial push-up fluidly before releasing the hands in the air.

- If you are ready to try the exercise but do not have much strength, you can minimize elbow flexion on the landing and minimize jump height. Just unload body weight from the hands. This results in a jump-shuffling of the hands out away from the ball.

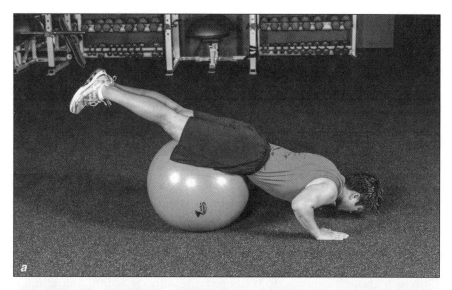

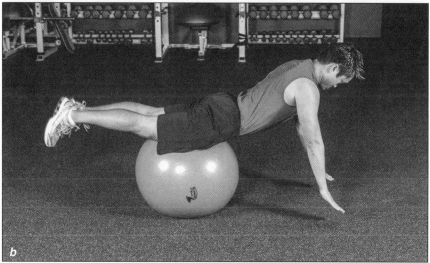

Jump Push-Up

This exercise develops braking and absorbing abilities that benefit powerful sport mechanics. The eccentric loading on an unstable surface improves muscle strength and reactivity in the core, shoulders, and posterior chain. Complete sets with the simplest demands and then progress to more difficult versions one step at a time. You must be able to complete multiple sets of ball balance push-ups and floor push-ups (feet on ball) before progressing to jump push-ups.

Setup

Prepare for the exercise by assuming a push-up position with feet on the floor shoulder-width apart and hands on the ball. The heel of the hand should rest on the outside upper portion of the ball with the fingers wrapped down around the ball. Set your core, load through the scapula, and press (squeeze) into the ball.

Movement

While remaining strong through the trunk and hips, lower the chest to the top of the ball, then extend the arms to push your body mass back to the top position. Push up with enough exertion to travel past the setup position, unloading your body mass from the ball.

Middle Position

At the middle position, land back onto the ball, catching your mass with good hand placement and slight elbow flexion. Try to brake and stop the movement as soon as possible.

Finish

After you land, catch, brake, and pause, resume lowering into another rep.

Tips and Progressions

- Spend extra time preparing for the exercise, ensuring you have set the core and upper back and have optimal body positioning, hand placement, and foot width.
- If you are new to this exercise, starting with a DSL ball will add stability to the landing.
- Spend time training at the following levels before advancing further:
  1. Push up to unload your body mass from the ball, releasing the heel of the hands but keeping fingers securely positioned on the ball. This provides the dynamic eccentric loading but reduces the load, skill, and balance required. Most active strength training enthusiasts can safely handle this level.
  2. Push off the ball until the full hand releases, producing as little height as possible.
  3. Push off higher, progressing the height over several workouts.

4. Add to the push-off jump height by also pulling the hands toward the trunk, maximizing the coordination and strength needed for absorbing the eccentric loading.

5. Revert to level 1 or 2 but land and catch with one hand only. Roll to two hands for the lowering and push-up phase, alternating arms on the catch.

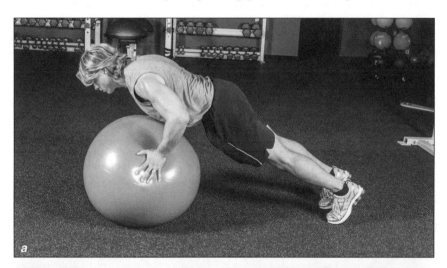

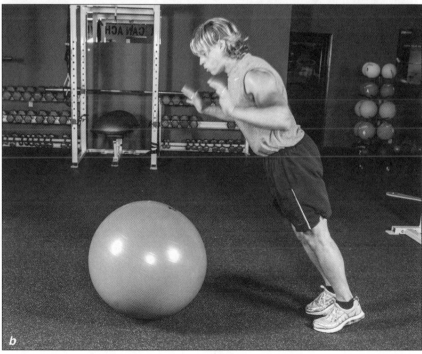

Standing Medicine Ball Press-Away

This exercise not only works the chest area of the shoulder but also ties in the significant requirement of core stabilization.

Setup

Stand approximately 3 to 4 feet (~1 m) from a wall. Place a medicine ball about 4 inches (10 cm) below the line from your shoulder, and hold the ball with an extended arm against the wall. You will need to be on your toes with your core engaged as you lean into the ball with your one arm. Do not allow any rotation in the core as you get into the setup position.

Movement

While maintaining stabilization of your core, eccentrically lower your body toward the wall. You must do this in a slow and controlled manner.

Finish

Once you have lowered yourself down to a point where your shoulder is almost in full extension, press back out, again in a controlled manner. This movement is not meant to be performed with a fast tempo.

Tips and Progressions

- To increase the difficulty of this exercise, decrease the base of support by using a smaller medicine ball.
- Try unilateral leg support by raising the leg opposite of the working arm.

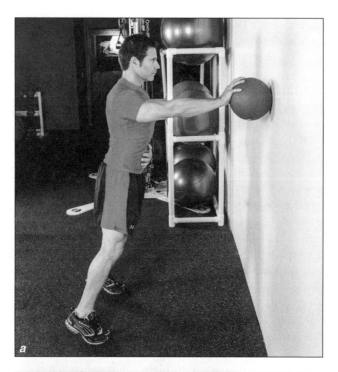

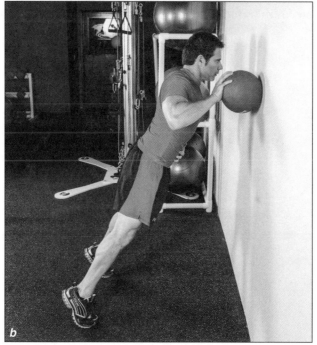

Ball Walk-Around

This is a great exercise for shoulder stabilization and core stability. The purpose is to load each shoulder independently.

Setup

Standing behind the ball, crouch down and place your abdominals on top of the ball. Roll forward until your hands reach the floor in front of the ball. Walk your hands out until your hips are off the ball. Continue to walk your hands out away from the ball until only your feet remain on the ball.

Movement

At this point, focus on maintaining a strong core and contracting the postural muscles to keep the hips up strong and body aligned. (Prevent the hips from sagging, and avoid any hip or torso rotation.) Maintaining a long lever (feet on the ball with body in a push-up position), walk your hands laterally to rotate your body around the ball in a clockwise direction. Pick up your right hand and move it away from your midline, supporting your body weight with your left arm until you replant the right hand. Next, pick up your left hand and move it in closer to the right hand. Alternate these steps so your hands complete a circle around the ball. Maintain a strong body alignment as you move your hands.

Finish

The movement is finished once you complete a 360-degree circle. Next, complete this pattern in a counterclockwise direction.

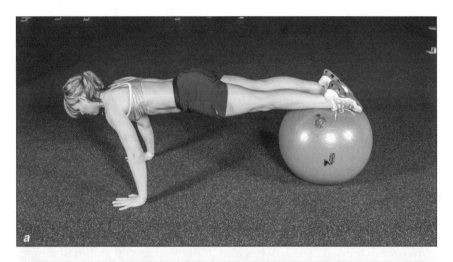

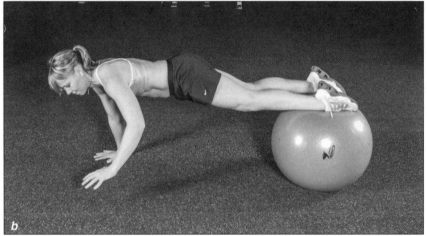

Medicine Ball Chest Pass

Chest passes link strength and power in the chest, shoulder, and back. The catch is absorbed with the core and legs. The return pass is initiated from the legs and hips and completed with the chest and arms. In its advanced form, it is an excellent full-body multijoint exercise.

Setup

Stand facing your partner, about three paces apart. Keep your feet shoulder-width apart, knees slightly flexed, and abdominals contracted. Both participants set up with the arms fully extended out level with the chest. The hands are open, making a definitive target.

Movement

Partner A draws the ball into the chest and reverses direction to push the ball out away from the body and onto partner B. Partner B first makes ball contact with the arms fully extended. The ball is sequentially absorbed through flexing of the arms and knees to cushion the catch. Partner B tries to overcome the eccentric loading as quickly as possible, immediately reversing direction to push the ball back toward partner A.

Finish

When you pass, after releasing the ball, keep your arms extended and up and out away from the chest, with an open hand target. Continue this sequence for a set number of repetitions.

Tips and Progressions

- For speed, complete the same exercise technique but position only two paces apart. Pass as quickly as possible, trying to eliminate any pause at the chest between the negative and positive phases of movement. Hand targets are important for protecting your face. Be positioned to maintain the rapid-pass succession.

- For strength, repeat the same exercise instruction, but five paces apart. Minimize the time between the negative phase and reverse direction into a positive push phase. This will be more challenging because the load you catch will be heavier with the extra distance. More full-body linked strength is needed for propelling the ball the required distance.

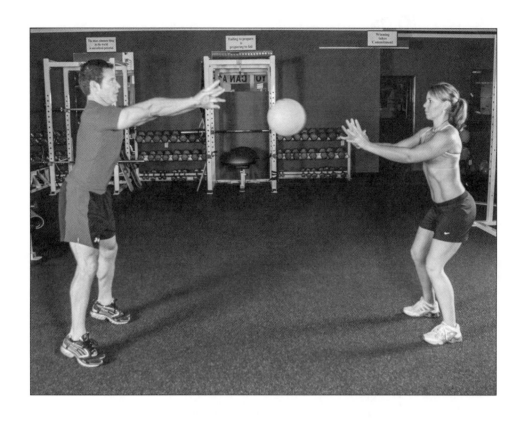

Standing Partner Stability Ball Chest Press

This exercise upgrades a push movement pattern into a closed kinetic chain position. Working with a partner, it begins with a focus on the eccentric phase linked with shoulder and core stabilization. After this preparatory work, it advances to a whole-body, multijoint push action.

Setup

Partners stand facing one another with the core braced, middle back set, and feet shoulder-width apart. The braking and stabilizing partner begins with arms fully extended; the pushing partner starts with arms flexed and ball at the chest.

Movement

One partner extends the arms to push the ball forward while the other slows the movement down, actively braking the force. Brace strongly to anchor the torso during the standing push. Likewise, maintain a set middle back so you do not compensate through the shoulders.

Finish

Once the ball is pushed through to the partner's chest, reverse roles and continue back and forth, alternating between pushing and braking.

Tips and Progressions

- Anyone with arms fully extended has the benefit of a locked lever system that is stronger than most muscular force. So to allow the partner to initiate the first rep, the braking and stabilizing partner may have to slightly flex at the elbows. To accommodate partners of unequal strength, the braking and stabilizing partner can ease up to allow the pushing partner to successfully extend the arms to a full range-of-motion push.

- After working on the exercise through several workouts and demonstrating solid posture and shoulder position during the braking action, advance to a multijoint push. In this version, before pushing, drop your center of mass by loading up the legs into a partial squat position. Focus on the sequential firing of muscles through the legs, hips, chest, and arms to first drive from the legs then push from the chest. This will require greater strength from the braking partner, who may now have to adopt a split stance to provide enough resistance.

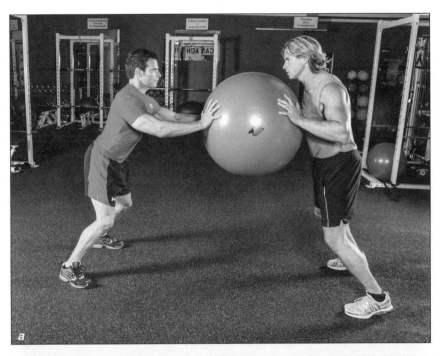

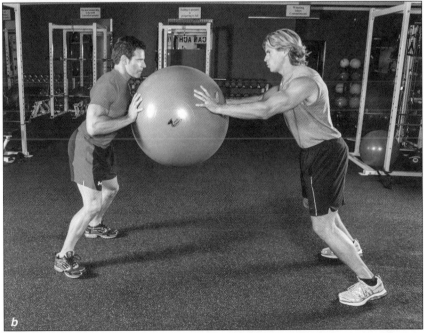

Dip With Medicine Ball or Stability Ball Squeeze

Dips are a great overall upper-body strength move. The ability to handle your own body weight is a great indicator of relative strength. Many people tend to flex their hips as they perform dips, thereby using some momentum to complete the movement. By squeezing a medicine ball or strength ball between the heels or the knees, you create a knee flexion movement to counteract the hips.

Setup

Begin in the top position of the dip and have a partner place a strength ball (no load) or a medicine ball (load) between your knees.

Movement

Before you begin your decent into the dip, squeeze your knees into the ball. Your knees should be pointing straight down toward the floor. Lower yourself to a point where your upper arms are parallel to the floor.

Finish

Without using any momentum, re-emphasize the ball squeeze and press back up to an extended position.

Tips and Progressions

This is a great method for teaching proper technique in the dip. As strength increases you may user a heavier medicine ball or add a weight vest.

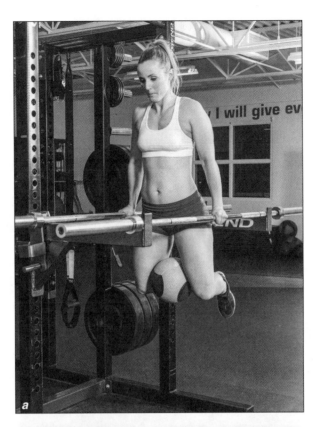

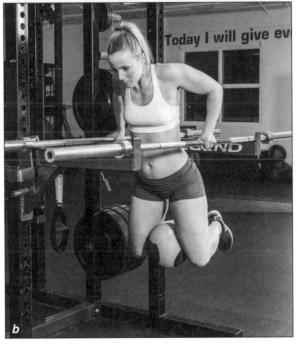

Strength Ball Decline Dumbbell Press

This decline press movement is a great way to hit the lower fibers of your pectorals. Most pressing movements focus on the middle and upper fibers.

Setup

Lying on the floor or a mat, grab two dumbbells and place your feet on top of a stability ball.

Movement

Engage your core and squeeze your glutes so your hips come off the floor. Keeping your core solid, lower your arms to a point where you feel your triceps just touch the floor.

Finish

Pause in the bottom position for a second or two and raise the dumbbells back to a fully extended position.

Tips and Progressions

Try using only one DB with an arm at your side to create an offset effect that will engage your core a bit more.

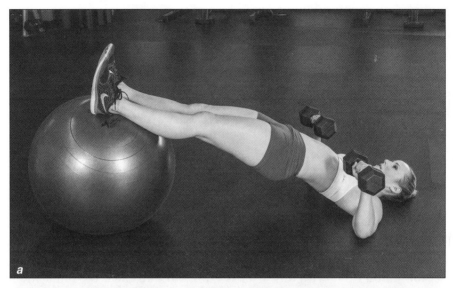

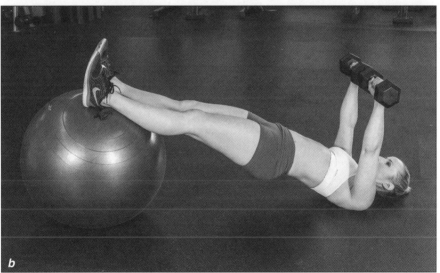

Supine Chest Push to Self-Catch

Self-catching throws bring a level of unpredictability to how the medicine ball loads on the body, requiring varied hand and arm position on the catch. This builds up joints, keeps muscles challenged and thinking, and asks the core to support the action.

Setup

Sit on the stability ball holding a medicine ball and walk out into a level supine bridge, hips up strong, and feet flat on the floor at shoulder width.

Movement

Push the ball up into the air away over the chest for maximum height. Fully extend the arms to express strength right through to the fingertips. Aim to still your torso and sustain raised hips during the throw and catch.

Finish

Catch the medicine ball with two hands, decelerating slowly to cushion the catch. Reset for another powerful throw rep. Be prepared to catch the medicine ball with two hands wherever it comes down. Less accurate throws mean an uneven bilateral push so the ball return may be either symmetrical or asymmetrical.

Tips and Progression

- To develop more eccentric strength, catch the ball by suddenly braking to specific joint angles.
- Switching to independent-arms catch and throw moves the ball back and forth, from left-hand catch to right-hand catch. Throws farther away from the body result in a fly-position catch, which can be incidental or a purposeful aim of the exercise execution.

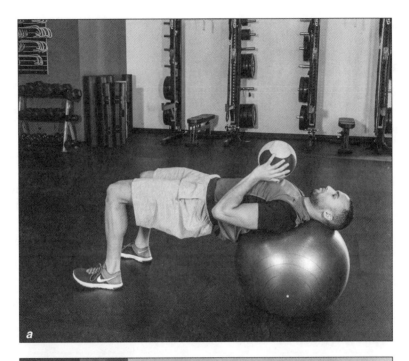

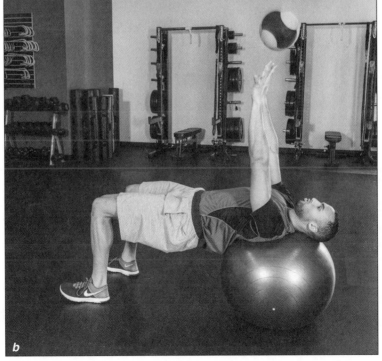

Push-Up Pass

This is a great upper-body plyometric exercise that prepares the body for eccentric loading and concentric power.

Setup

Partners are two strides apart, both kneeling on a folded sit-up mat. Torso is upright. One partner has a medicine ball.

Movement

Partner A (who has the ball) begins the drill by passing chest to chest to his partner. The arms remain extended out and the torso follows the pass, falling forward until the hands make contact on the floor and absorb the body into a push-up position. Powerfully push back up to reverse the direction and propel the torso back up into a kneeling position. On the way back up, as soon as both partners make eye contact, partner B returns the pass back to partner A and falls into a push-up position.

Finish

Continue this sequence for a set number of reps or until fatigue prevents pushing back up to a kneeling position. Especially as you fatigue and the tempo slows and decision making becomes inhibited, remember to wait for eye contact before returning passes.

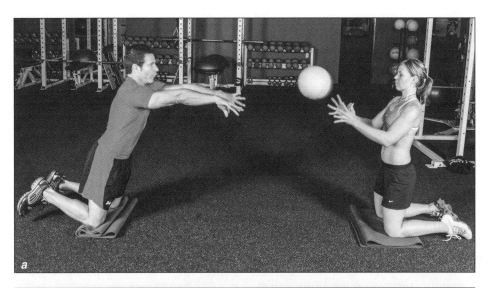

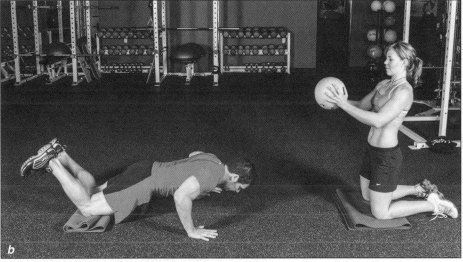

One-Arm Dumbbell Press

This exercise integrates anterior deltoids, pectorals, and core stabilization with a unilateral lift.

Setup

Sit on the stability ball with a dumbbell in one hand. Walk out so that you are in a supine position with your head and shoulders supported on the ball and feet at shoulder-width stance. Activate the core and glutes to keep the hips up and stable on the ball. Start with the entire dumbbell outside the shoulder.

Movement

The concentric movement will begin similar to a bench press action: Push the weight up on an arc, finishing above the shoulder.

Middle Position

In the middle of the rep, the arm is fully extended. Maintain a strong supine bridge with the glutes firing to keep the hips up level with knees and trunk. Shoulders remain on top of the ball.

Finish

Slowly lower the dumbbell under control, out and down, back to the setup position outside the shoulder. Bringing the load outside the midline will accelerate the demands for the core to stabilize the body position.

Tips and Progressions

- To progress, alternately increase the weight and decrease the base of support by bringing the feet closer together. Decreasing the base of support increases core activation while increasing the weight on the pecs and shoulders.

- If prime mover strength is your goal, to integrate some instability but prioritize the load imposed on the muscles, set up with a DSL stability ball and use a wide base of support, which allows you to use a heavier dumbbell.

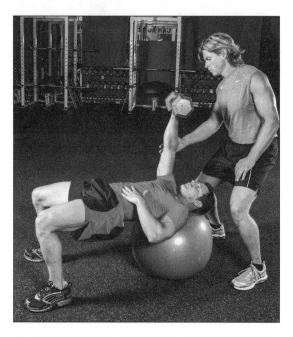

Standing–Lying Partner Push-Up and Press

This exercise develops less power than the standing partner chest press but is excellent for strength and joint stability. It capitalizes on the muscle reactivity needed for accommodating the shifting ball as the partner tries to hold it.

Setup

Partner A lies faceup on the floor with knees flexed, feet flat on the floor, and core set. Partner B stands up in front of partner A's feet. Facing each other, they hold a stability ball between them with the heels of their hands on the ball and fingers wrapping down around the sides of the ball. Elbows are only slightly flexed. Partner B stands with flexed knees, weight leaning into the ball.

Movement

Partner A flexes the arms to slowly lower the ball (and partial weight of partner) to the chest before pressing back up. During this movement, partner B pivots on the toes to travel with the ball as it is lowered. The goal for partner B is to stabilize on the ball, maintaining a straight line from heel to shoulder.

Partner A next presses into the ball, extending the arms to push the ball back up (against partner B's body weight). This relies on partner B to isometrically contract to hold the ball in place during the movement.

Finish

After partner A pushes the ball back up to the setup position, partner B lowers into the ball and then pushes back up, relying on partner A to isometrically contract to hold the ball in place.

Tips and Progressions

- Give each partner sets in both positions.
- An advanced challenge is for partner A to slightly shift the ball left and right during his push-up, challenging partner B to maintain a locked system from heel to trunk while the ball is being lowered and raised.

CHAPTER 8

SHOULDERS AND UPPER BACK

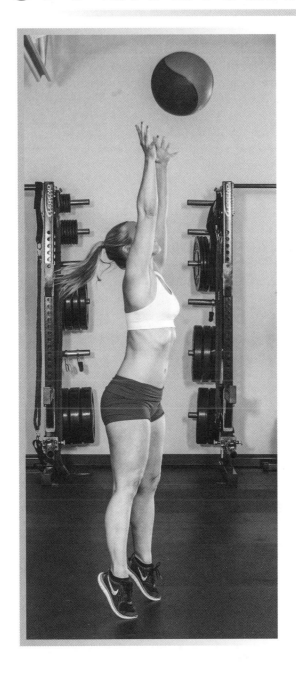

Prone Row External Rotation

The goal of the prone row external rotation is to integrate two functional movements into one exercise. Recruitment of the extensor muscles of the entire spine is also emphasized during this exercise.

Setup

Place the stability ball under your middle chest and align your body so that your knees, hips, shoulders, and neck are in a neutral aligned position as demonstrated in the setup position.

Movement

With your hands holding dumbbells in an extended position under the shoulders, pull your elbows directly up, ensuring that your upper arms are in a straight line across your body. If you were viewing this from the top, you could draw a straight line from elbow to elbow, right across the upper back. The elbows should never rise above this horizontal line. If you have problems with shoulder impingement, you should find a comfortable range of motion slightly below this position to ease any potential shoulder pain.

Finish

Once you bring your elbows up, stabilize this position and externally rotate your upper arms. Maintain a 90-degree angle at the elbow joint, which will guarantee a longer lever and ensure optimal loading of the external rotator musculature. Rotate to the point where your upper and lower arm are in a horizontal position with the floor, as demonstrated in the finish position. Hold this position for one second and then derotate. Lower arms to the start position and repeat for a set number of reps.

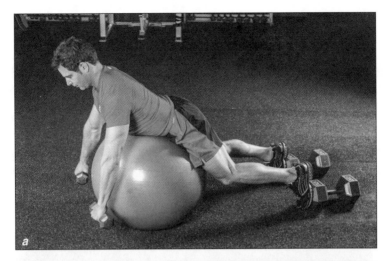

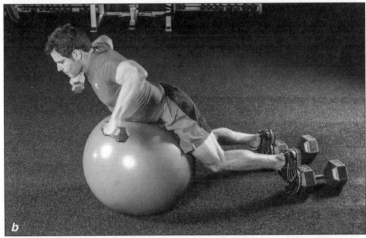

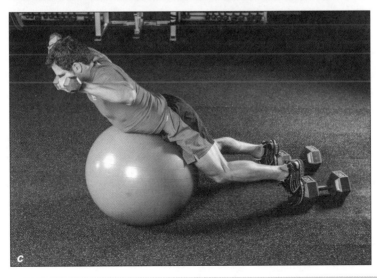

Cross-Body Rear Delt Raise

This exercise targets the important muscles in the back of the shoulders that help to stabilize the shoulder blades. The position in which you place your body will also challenge your core muscles.

Setup

Lie sideways over the ball, with the ball placed in your armpit and on the side of your chest. Maintain this lateral position throughout the movement.

Movement

Set your abdominals and draw in your navel. With your arm extended and pointing toward the floor holding a dumbbell, begin to raise your arm away from your body.

Finish

As you continue to raise your arm, your core will be challenged to stabilize your body on the ball. Continue to maintain a good position on the ball. Bring your arm up to the point where it is 5 degrees before perpendicular. At this point, hold the position for two seconds, and lower the arm to the setup position for your next rep.

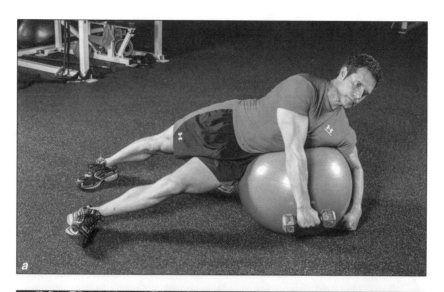

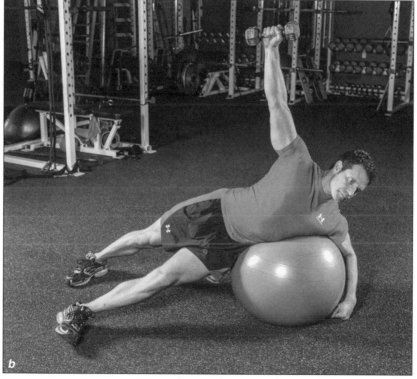

Reverse Tubing Fly

The reverse fly stresses the shoulder through a large range of motion. The single-arm cross-body line of pull challenges the core to stabilize trunk and ball position.

Setup

Sitting on the stability ball, walk the feet out away from the ball until you achieve a supine bridge position: head and shoulder blades on the ball, back and hips parallel to the floor. Attach one end of the tubing to something solid such as a door frame or piece of exercise equipment. Hold the other handle of strength tubing across the body, with a prestretch on the strength tubing.

Movement

Keeping the elbow slightly flexed, pull the handle up and over your body in an arc.

Middle Position

In mid-rep, hips are up and trunk remains strong. With light tubing, the handle should end up level with the shoulder. With stronger resistance, stop above the shoulder for an isometric hold.

Finish

Bring the handle back over the body with a controlled pace, providing active resistance against the shortening tubing.

Tips and Progressions

- To regress, select lighter tubing or position the ball closer to where the other end of the strength tubing is fixed, but be sure to have a prestretch on the tubing at the setup position.
- Progress the drill with stronger tubing and slower movement on both the concentric (positive) and eccentric (negative) phases.
- For greater emphasis on shoulder strength, use heavier tubing and a wider base of support at the feet.
- For more core emphasis, use moderate tubing with a narrow base of support.

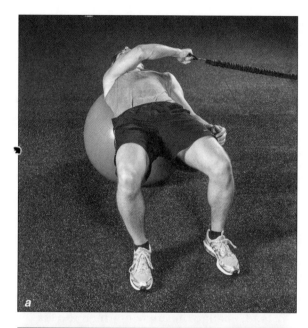

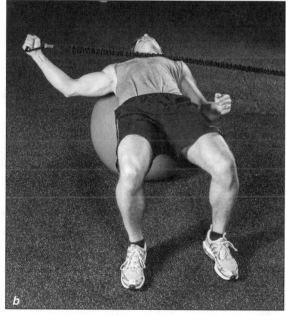

Isodynamic Rear Delt Raise

This is unique because it incorporates isometric exercise (muscle contraction with no movement) and movement all within a single exercise. The targeted muscles surround the shoulder, shoulder blade, neck extensors, and spinal extensors.

Setup

Lie prone on the ball, with the ball placed just below your chest. Your body should be positioned so that the ankles, knees, and hips are in line and the torso is flexed forward so your upper body is at about a 45-degree angle with the floor. With a dumbbell in each hand and while maintaining the setup position, raise your arms until they are almost parallel to the floor.

Movement

Once your arms are in the proper position, there is actually no movement. This is the isometric type of contraction. Hold this position for 5 to 10 seconds. Maintain good head posture during this effort.

Finish

After 5 to 10 seconds, you will find that the shoulder musculature tires quite quickly. To ease the load, change the angle at which the load is placed on your shoulders. Bend your knees and roll back on the ball approximately 20 degrees. Maintain the same posture and arm position. Once you have rolled back, you will be able to hold position for another 5 to 10 seconds. The set is now completed. Lower the dumbbells to the floor, and rest for the prescribed time.

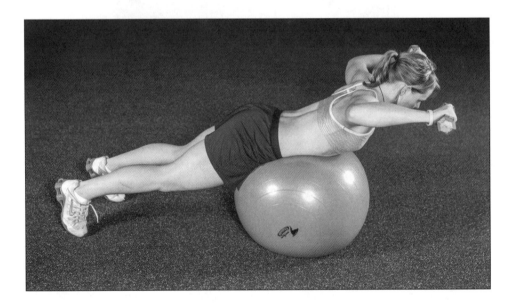

Supine Lat Pull and Delt Raise

This exercise focuses on training the contralateral muscles, which involves training the latissimus dorsi on the posterior side of one shoulder while training the anterior deltoid on the opposite shoulder.

Setup

With a dumbbell in each hand, sit on a stability ball and roll out so you are in a tabletop position. One arm should be in extension—the upper arm is in line with the ear—and the other arm is in a neutral position by the hip. Use a neutral grip. Activate the glutes and core to provide a stable base for movement.

Movement

Begin by flexing the extended arm; at the same time extend the opposite side. Both arms begin the movement in unison. Keep the glutes and core activated to maintain a stable base for movement.

Finish

Your arms will be in the opposite position to that of the starting position.

Tips and Progressions

- By changing your hand position from a neutral grip to palms facing the ceiling, you place a greater challenge on the latissimus dorsi in the overhead position. This is a result of the internal rotation at the shoulder that will change the grip. The lats are also an internal rotator.

- To increase the activity of the core and glutes, you can place a weight vest or sandbag over the abdominals.

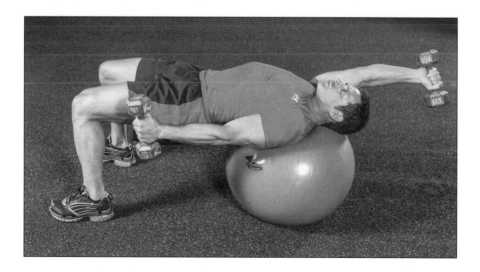

Pullover

The pullover is an excellent move that will help anyone who lacks overhead shoulder extension. This exercise takes your pectoral muscles and latissimus dorsi through a complete range of motion.

Setup

With a dumbbell in each hand, sit on a stability ball and roll out so you are in a tabletop position. The ball should support your head and shoulders. Extend both arms so that your biceps are in line with your ears.

Movement

Flex your arms forward to a position where they are straight up at a 90-degree angle with your body.

Finish

Lower your arms back to the starting position and repeat.

Tips and Progressions

- Keep your core engaged and do not arch your back as you lower your arms down to the extended position.
- You can also alternate arms so that each one moves independently.

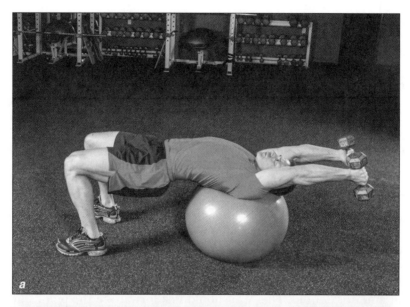

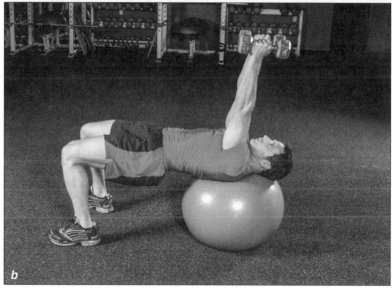

Prone Front Raise Lateral Fly

The prone front raise lateral fly fires up your whole posterior chain with a major emphasis on the shoulder adductors and extensors. Coordination between the left and right sides of the body will be put to the test.

Setup

Depending on your type of floor, it may be advantageous to set up near a wall. Brace both feet against the base of the floor and wall while placing the stability ball just above your navel. Your head, shoulders, hips, and knees should form a fairly straight line at approximately 45 degrees. Holding dumbbells in both hands, your arms should be extended under your chest.

Movement

Engage your core before the shoulders fire. The left arm begins extending out to the side as a lateral fly, challenging your rhomboids and posterior deltoid. Bring this arm up to the point where it is in line with your body and parallel to the floor. You should be able to draw a line across your back, connecting your scapula with your elbow. At the same time your right arm will flex forward as you fire your anterior deltoid. This arm should flex forward to the point where it is in line with your head and parallel to the floor.

Finish

Once you have reached the contracted positions, hold them for a second or two. This will result in a stability and balance effort of your upper torso. After you pause, return to the starting position and reverse the movement. Now the left arm will flex forward and the right arm will extend out to the side.

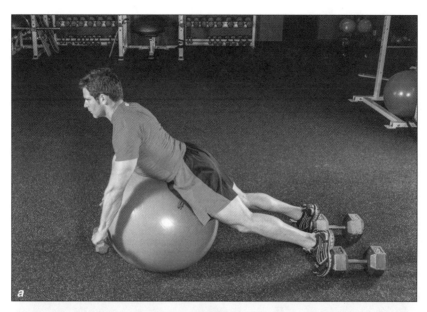

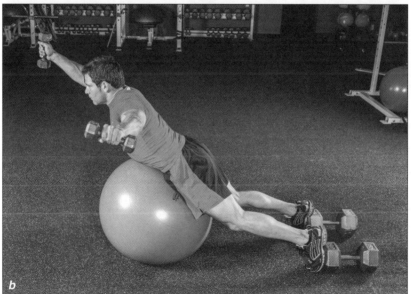

Supine Pull-Up

The supine pull-up is a great overall exercise for all muscles on the back side of the body. It requires postural muscles to fire to keep the body in proper alignment while the shoulders pull the body up and down.

Setup

Set yourself up in a power rack so that the height of the barbell will allow for full extension of your arms without allowing your upper back to touch the floor. Your grip determines which muscles will be emphasized. An overhand grip with your elbows pointing outward directs more resistance to the posterior deltoid and rhomboids. An underhand grip with your elbows pointing inward emphasizes the latissimus dorsi. The grip should be shoulder width or slightly narrower for the underhand grip.

Begin with the stability ball under the knees. As you become stronger, you will progress by moving the ball toward your heels. The size of your ball will dictate how hard the exercise will be. Begin with a smaller ball; as you become stronger, progress to a larger ball.

Movement

Before you begin to pull yourself up, ensure that your knees, hips, and shoulders are in line. The muscles in your hips and back should be precontracted to stabilize your body into this position. Avoid tucking your chin in to view your body. You should be looking at the ceiling, with your head in a neutral position.

As you begin your movement, pull yourself up to the point where you can touch your chest to the bar. As you reach this position, attempt to squeeze your shoulder blades together to emphasize the muscles between your shoulder blades and spine.

Finish

As your chest touches the bar, hold this position for two seconds, and lower yourself to the start position. Allow yourself to get a good stretch in your upper back, then repeat.

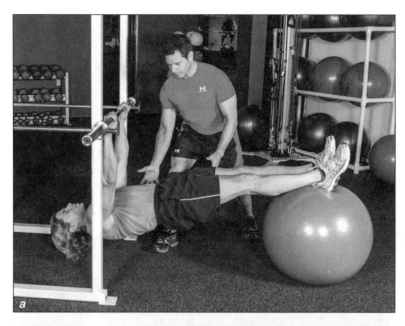

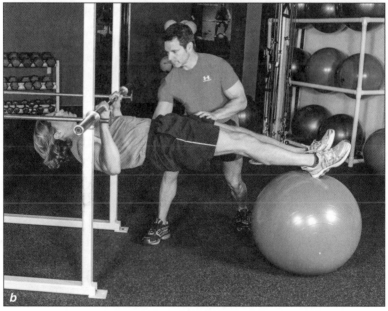

Seated Rotator Cuff Pull

With so many great push exercises and lateral shoulder moves, special attention is required for the posterior chain. You enjoy the most versatile range of motion in the shoulder joint, but to balance out shoulder mobility, strength is needed. Rotator cuff exercises will help build a stronger shoulder base, equalizing the push and lateral strength. Strengthening the rotator cuff muscle group will also improve your ability to set the middle back by using force closure to anchor the shoulders before any strength maneuver.

Setup

Sit on the stability ball facing the strength tubing axis point, which you affix at floor level around a column or at home with a door attachment. Brace the core and set the upper back. Sit up tall on the ball with good posture and feet shoulder-width apart on the floor. Knees should be level or just below hip height. Holding the tubing or cable, your arm is in an abducted position with a 90-degree bend in the elbow.

Movement

Keeping the elbow up, pull the strength tubing up and back until the elbow is in line with and level to the shoulder. Keep pulling the tubing by rotating around the elbow. The elbow remains fixed while the hand moves up and over the elbow.

Middle Position

In mid-rep, your elbow remains level with the shoulder, hand above the shoulder, and trunk perpendicular to the line of pull.

Finish

Slowly lower the tubing under control, reversing the two movement phases. Rotate around the elbow until the hand is level with the elbow and shoulder, then release and extend the arm under control.

Tips and Progressions

- A common error is trunk rotation to assist the pull. If the trunk does not stay square to the line of pull, remove the ball and practice this exercise in a standing position (on the floor), or select lighter tubing that the rotator cuff muscles can handle without assistance from the trunk.
- To increase the complexity and core activation, perform the exercise while kneeling on the ball.

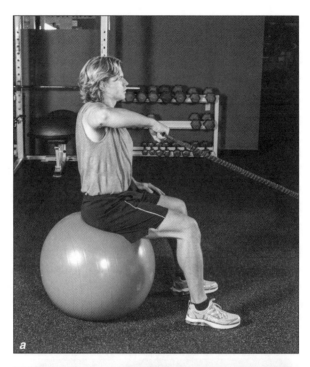

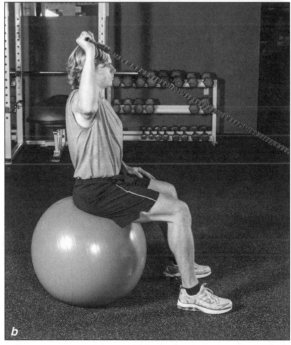

Medicine Ball Push Press

This is an explosive movement that enhances full-body explosive vertical power with an emphasis on the deltoids. You will need a heavier ball and a higher ceiling for this exercise.

Setup

Get set in an athletic position, hips back, knees slightly bent, and ankles flexed, holding a medicine ball at shoulder height.

Movement

Very quickly drop your hips to a quarter-squat position, keeping your core engaged and your body solid. To begin the upward movement, you want to change your direction as fast as you can as you begin to explode upward.

Finish

As you are moving toward full-body extension, you should move your arms upward with the medicine ball to continue the upward acceleration, releasing the ball when you are fully extended. Let the ball fall to the floor; do not try to catch it and repeat.

Tips and Progressions

Attempt to release the ball at your highest point.

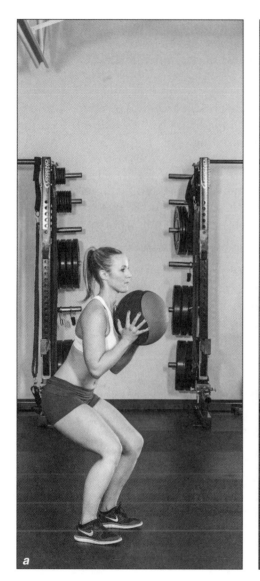

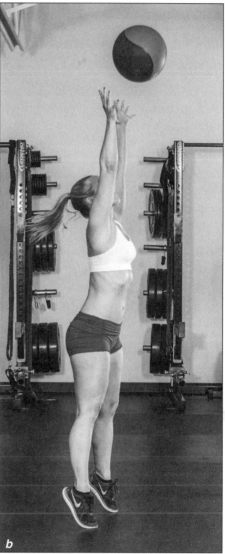

Prone Medicine Ball Transfer

The prone medicine ball transfer works a combination of mobility and strength through a full range of motion in the shoulder. Most important, it works many upper-back muscles that help support the whole shoulder girdle.

Setup

In a prone position on the floor, place your neck in a neutral position with your chin tucked in. Start by holding one small medicine ball on one side with the palm pronated so your palm is toward the ceiling.

Movement

Engage your core so you can maintain a neutral spine and begin to bring your arm up and around toward your head. Midway through the movement on the one side, begin to pronate your hand so by the time your arm reaches the full extension over your head, your palm is facing down.

Finish

As your first arm movement reaches extension, you will meet it with the opposite arm, hand the ball off in a prone hand position, and repeat the movement on the opposite side. As you come around, though, you will pass the ball off behind your back.

Tips and Progressions

- Reverse the direction with each set or after completing half the reps within a set.
- Do not allow your spine to go into extension as you begin to fatigue.
- Use higher repetitions and lighter ball weights to maximize the postural capabilities of these muscles.

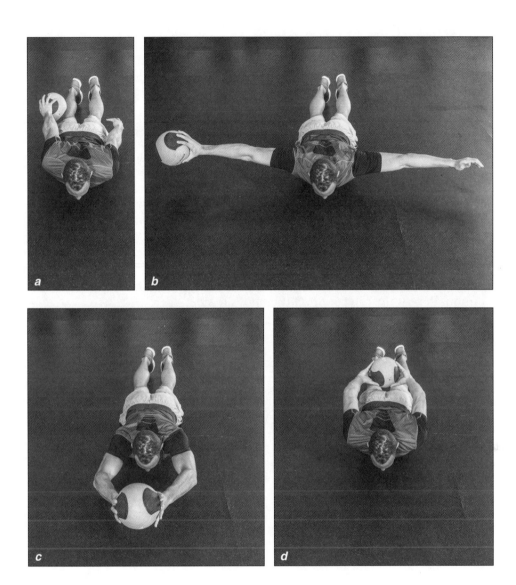

Medicine Ball Athletic-Ready Unilateral Wall Press

Holding a ball against the wall applies force perpendicular to the line of travel, loading the posterior chain preferentially.

Setup

Begin facing away from a wall in a tall athletic-ready stance with the core engaged and the back of one hand pressing into a medicine ball to hold it in place.

Movement

Anchoring the legs and torso in place, extend the arm overhead, keeping pressure on the ball as your hand rolls the ball up the wall. Reach as high as your strength permits.

Finish

Pull from the upper back to initiate the drawing of the ball back down to setup position. Repeat the rep count on the opposite side.

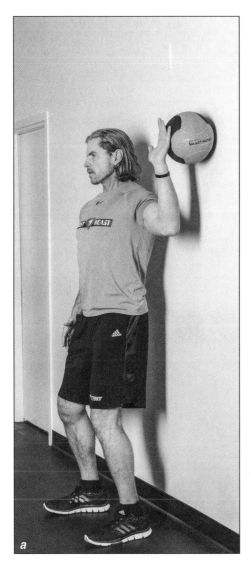
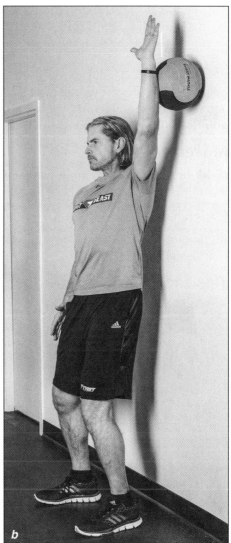

Medicine Ball Squat-Away Posterior Chain Wall Hold

This begins at the strongest joint angle where using a weighted ball will be difficult, demanding significant strength along the kinetic chain from hand along to glutes, pressuring with the posterior chain.

Setup

Begin facing away from a wall in a tall athletic-ready stance with the core engaged and the back of one hand pressing into a medicine ball to hold it in place. Position the ball so the hand is shoulder height, elbow toward waist.

Movement

Hold the medicine ball in the same location the entire rep. Drop the body away from the ball by lowering into a deep squat, leaving the arm extended overhead.

Finish

Initiate the return back to a standing position with the upper back, not just the rear shoulders.

Tips and Progressions

- Sustain pressure against the ball at all times.
- If the ball begins to roll or falls to the floor, reset where you paused in that rep and continue.

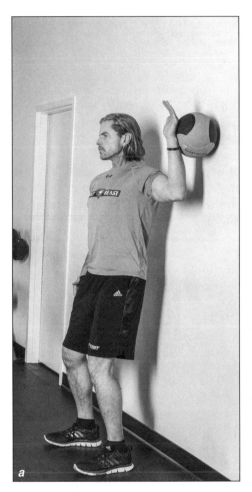
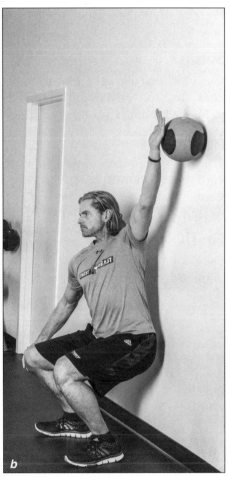

Scapular Pull

Most shoulder problems are a result of weak musculature on the posterior side of the shoulder and in the muscles that span from the spine over the scapula. This exercise strengthens those muscles and provides balance between the stronger muscles in the front of the shoulder to those in the back.

Setup

Use a ball that allows your arms to be in the fully extended position toward the floor while you are holding dumbbells. With dumbbells in hand, lie over the ball so the ball is under your sternum. Your shoulders, hips, and knees fall in line.

Movement

Contract the muscles of your lower trapezius so that your scapulae slide downward toward your rib cage. This movement can be described as depressing your shoulders. As you reach the end range for your scapulae, begin to externally rotate your hands to further work these muscles.

Finish

Once you have fully externally rotated your shoulders, hold this position for two to three seconds and return to the start position.

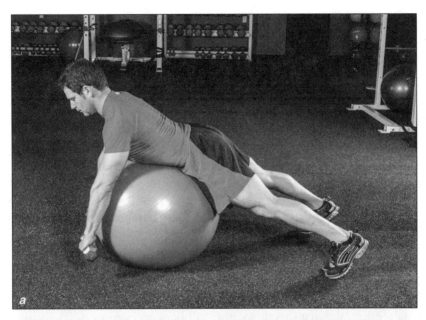

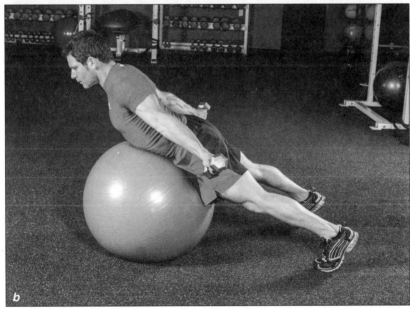

Medicine Ball Shoulder-to-Shoulder Pass

This drill develops strength in the shoulder and back region and links the strength through the legs, hips, torso, and upper body. In its advanced forms, balance, proprioception, and countermovement mechanics are all emphasized.

Setup

Stand facing your partner, about three paces apart. Keep your feet shoulder-width apart, knees slightly flexed, and abdominals contracted.

Movement

Partner A positions a hand and the medicine ball directly in front of the right shoulder. The pass line goes from the right shoulder to partner B's right shoulder. Partner B prepares to receive the ball by flexing the knees, contracting the core, and fully extending the arms, giving the partner a target. The goal is to cushion the pass reception with the entire body. The ball comes into the hands and the arms bend, drawing in the ball closer to the right shoulder. The hips drop and the body weight shifts onto the right leg, flexing at the knee. This is a whole-body catch. The pass back reverses the flow. The pass begins by pushing the foot into the floor, extending the leg, rotating with the hip and torso, and finally extending the arms to thrust the ball back to partner A. The arm movement is more of a direct push from the shoulder (similar to a shot put) rather than a throw in baseball.

Finish

Continue this sequence for a set number of repetitions. Repeat the set from left shoulder to left shoulder.

Tips and Progressions

- One-arm shoulder-to-shoulder pass: Execute the same technique and progression with one arm only. To catch the ball, you will rely more on absorbing and cushioning the ball with your entire body. It becomes a torso and lower-body catch. You will also rely on the quality of the pass. When first attempting this advanced exercise, your partner will tend to lob a soft and arced pass, which is difficult to catch. A crisp, straight pass from shoulder to shoulder will be easier to cushion and balance.

- One-arm and opposite-leg shoulder-to-shoulder pass: Follow the same exercise instruction but balance on one leg only. For the pass from right shoulder to right shoulder, both partners balance on the left leg. Superior balance, proprioception, core and hip stabilization, and multijoint pass reception are all challenged.

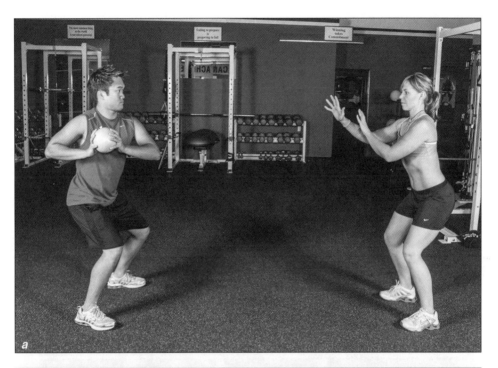

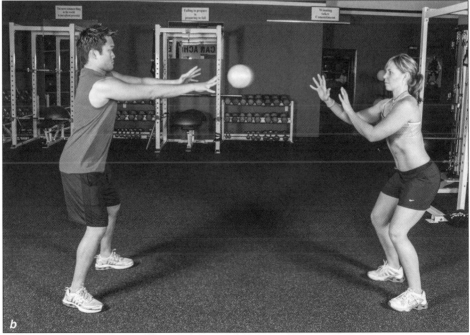

Scapular Push-Up

Two important muscles in the shoulder are the subscapularis and the serratus anterior. These muscles keep the shoulder blade against the rib cage during pressing movements. Scapular push-ups are an effective method of working this area.

Setup

Standing behind the ball, place your hands on the ball at shoulder width. Shuffle your feet back until your chest is over the ball and you are supported on your toes.

Movement

The movement is similar to that of regular push-ups. The difference is that the elbows do not flex and extend. All movement comes from a pushing movement out of the shoulder. This pushing movement creates a hunchback shape.

Finish

After pushing up to the point where you cannot push anymore, slowly lower yourself and allow your shoulder blades to come together without bending your elbows.

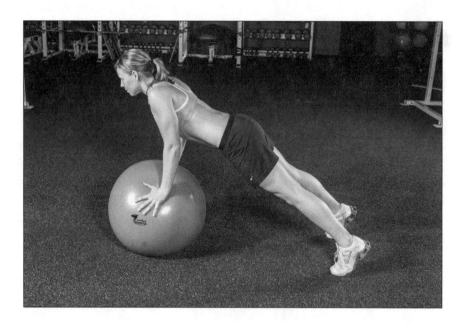

CHAPTER 9

ABDOMINALS, LOWER BACK, AND GLUTES

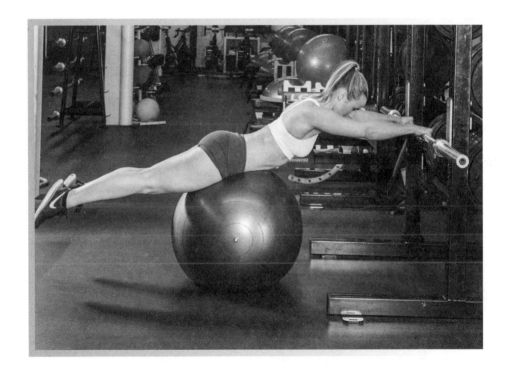

Wrap Sit-Up

This exercise is borrowed from traditional floor-based sit-ups. Refined technique is required so that you can feel the same burn in the abs that you would with floor-based crunches and sit-ups. Ball wrap sit-ups deliver superior strength results because the shape of the ball allows safe torso wrapping to prestretch the abdominals, allowing them to work through a greater range of motion. The shape of the ball is more comfortable on the back and better targets abdominals instead of firing hip flexors.

Setup

The setup position is key to the concentric contraction achieved at the peak of the sit-up. Sit on top of the ball and roll forward slightly. Feet are on the floor, shoulder-width apart. The setup is actually positioned at the midpoint of the exercise because its accuracy determines the level of abdominal overload achieved. When you sit up on the ball, you should hold a contraction and have the low back off the ball.

Movement

After setting the core, slowly lower, under control, onto the ball and continue to wrap right over the ball. Lower under control to work the eccentric muscle contraction. Avoid clasping hands behind the head. Instead, just make sure the arms are "quiet," whether they are crossed on your chest or flexed at your side. Keep them stationary through the movement to remove any momentum.

Middle Position

At the midpoint, pause at the end of the eccentric loading and sense the stretch before initiating movement back up and off the ball. Although you are actually only slightly wrapped around the ball, your perception is that you are almost upside down.

Finish

Slowly lift your trunk up off of the ball, segment by segment, until you are sitting upright, resting on your glutes.

Tips and Progressions

- Adopting a wider base of support can make this exercise easier.
- Advance the level of difficulty by placing your feet together, which requires greater muscle activation to stabilize on the ball during movement than does the wider base of support.
- After successful training with a narrow base, close your eyes to increase the demands. Any time you sense a loss of balance, open your eyes.

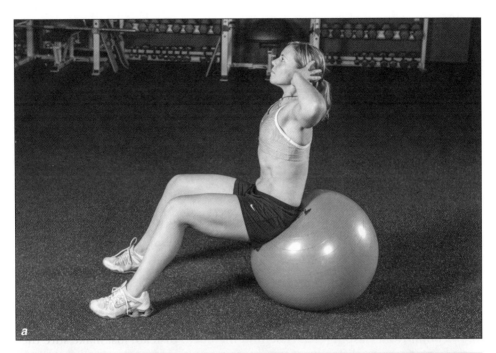

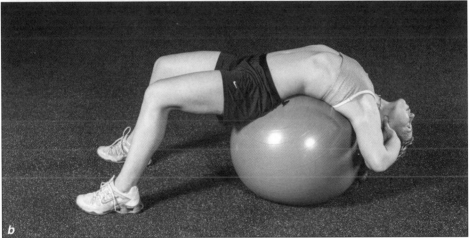

Adam's Medicine Ball Ab Lockout

This exercise was developed by Adam Douglas, a strength coach at the Athletic Conditioning Center. It is an excellent move that requires a partner. The exercise fires your rectus abdominis muscle. The key is not only the abdominal work but also the tie-in of the adductors to hold on to the medicine ball. This is an excellent method of integrating muscles in both the frontal plane and sagittal plane.

Setup

Lie on your back with your legs up in a 90-degree angle and your fingers touching your temples. Squeeze a medicine ball between your knees. Your elbows should be in contact with your thighs.

Movement

Once you are in this position, hold your elbows tight to your thighs. A partner grabs onto your knees and pulls you forward.

Finish

As you are pulled forward, stay very tight. Do not let your elbows come off your thighs.

Tips and Progressions

- To increase the difficulty of this exercise, your partner can use a faster and slower speed of rocking your body.
- The pull should never be explosive, just a controlled motion.

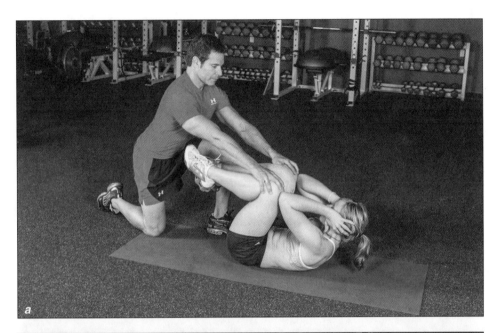

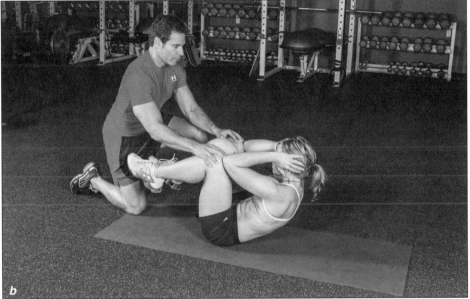

Supine Lower-Abdominal Cable Curl

This is an effective method of adding resistance to the lower-abdominal muscles. This area is key in controlling pelvic positioning, which can play a factor in decreasing low back pain.

Setup

Lying on the floor, with your legs over the ball, place a cable with an ankle strap around your ankles. Your hands should be under your lower back, at the navel level. Make sure that your back maintains contact with your hands. This ensures proper low back posture during the exercise.

Movement

Set your core and bring your knees toward your chest. Focus on not allowing your back to arch off the floor as you bring your knees up and back.

Finish

Once you have reached a point where your legs are just past the 90-degree point, slowly return to the start position.

Safety Note

If you cannot maintain your posture with the added load of the cable, then you should focus on performing the movement without the cable, progress to a medicine ball between your legs, and then try the cable again.

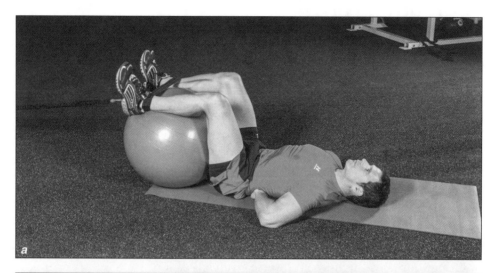

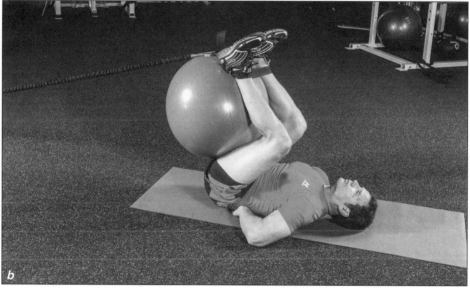

Supine Lower-Abdominal Curl and Crunch

This is the most advanced lower-abdominal exercise you will perform. It focuses on pelvic strength, stability, and balance.

Setup

Set a ball in front of something solid you can hold on to. The side of a power rack or a loaded barbell will do. Lie over the ball so that your lower back is supported by the curve of the ball and your knees are bent. Hold on to a rack overhead to stabilize yourself.

Movement

Begin by setting your core, and focus on uncurling your pelvis off of the curve of the ball. You will accomplish this by slowly bringing your knees toward you. As your legs reach the 90-degree point, try to touch the ceiling with your knees by lifting your pelvis higher in a reverse crunch position.

Finish

Once you have reached up as high as you can, hold that position for two to three seconds, then slowly return to the start position by reversing your movements.

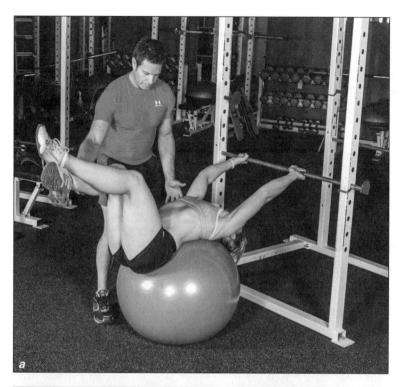

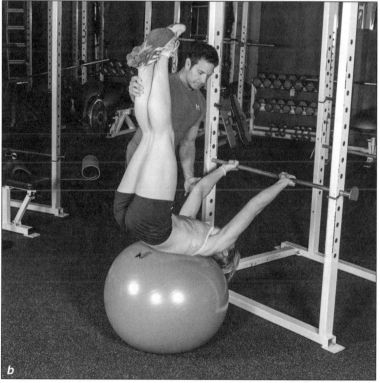

V-Sit Medicine Ball Transfer

This exercise challenges the core through a range of motion from extension to core flexion.

Setup

Lie on your back with arms fully extended over your head holding a medicine ball.

Movement

Begin by engaging your core and flexing at the waist. This will cause your legs and arms to rise at the same time. Flex forward until you can transfer the medicine ball from your hands to your feet.

Finish

Once you have transferred the ball to your feet, lower back to the starting position and repeat.

Tips and Progressions

- Ensure that as you flex forward your arms remain extended overhead.
- This exercise is quite advanced and challenging. You might want to begin with transferring a stability ball before progressing to a medicine ball.

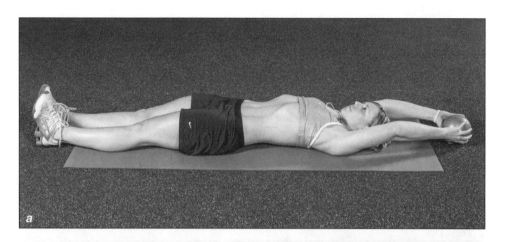

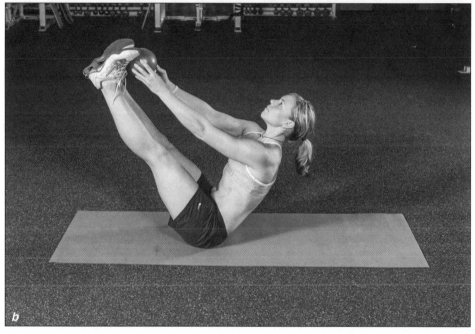

Reverse Back Extension

This exercise works the lower back. It uses both a ball and a bench, and the difficulty can be increased by using a cable attached to the ankles.

Setup

Place a stability ball on top of a flat bench, and lie over the ball while grasping the sides of the bench for support.

Movement

Begin by setting your core before attempting to extend the hips and legs. Your head and neck should also maintain a neutral position. Just before you begin to extend your hips and legs, activate the glutes by squeezing them to ensure that they initiate the movement.

Finish

The legs should be raised to a point where the knees, hips, and shoulders are all in line. Hold the contracted position for a second, and lower to the original position.

Tips and Progressions

You can slowly work up to the reverse hyperextension as the end of a long, safe progression. The following are some examples:

- Begin with the ball on the floor and hands braced on the floor for balance. Extend the hips. Begin with an underinflated ball, and progress to full inflation.

- Place the ball on a bench and perform movement with no external resistance. Begin with an underinflated ball, and progress to full inflation.

- Hold a 5- to 10-pound dumbbell (or 2.5 to 5 kg) between the ankles, and extend the hips.

- Progress to full reverse hyperextension with cable.

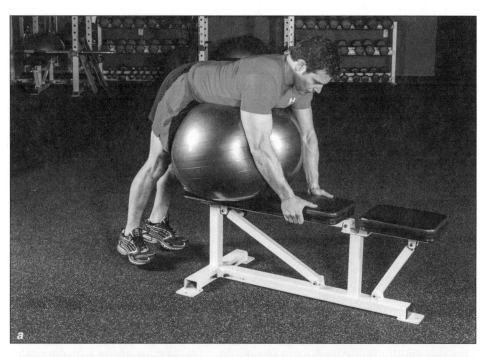

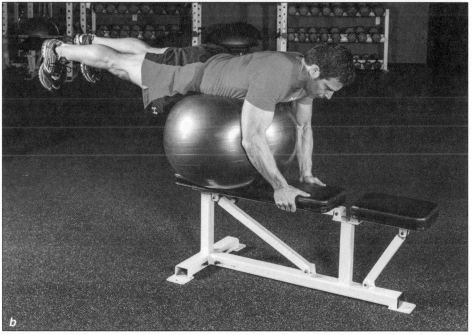

Back Extension

The back extension is an important movement in integrating the low back, glutes, and hamstrings. This exercise has been traditionally performed on a back extension bench. The stability ball allows for training in balance.

Setup

Place a stability ball in front of you, and lie over it. Your center of gravity should be just slightly behind the center of the ball. When starting out, ensure that your legs are wide enough apart to provide a good base of support to initiate the movement.

Movement

Place your hands by your ears, set your abdominals, activate your glutes, and slowly rise to the point at which your shoulders, hips, and knees are in a fairly straight line. Hold this position.

Finish

Slowly lower yourself back to the initial position, providing a stretch to your low back.

Tips and Progressions

- Bring legs closer together, decreasing your base of support and increasing the stability factor.
- Hold arms out straight with thumbs pointing to the ceiling (as in a superman pose) to increase the lever arm length and stress to the back and glutes.

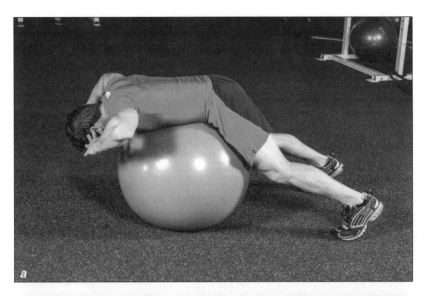

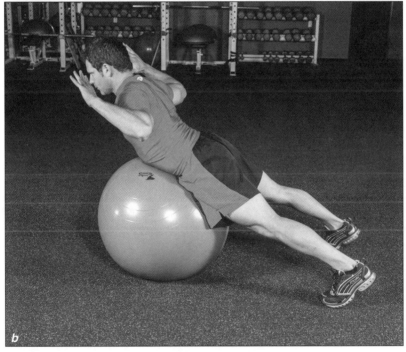

Barbell Hip Extension
With Medicine Ball Squeeze

This exercise ties in the glutes with the hip adductors, turning it into a multiplanar lower-body challenge.

Setup

Lying on your back, bring a loaded barbell over your hips. You may need a foam pad under the bar; otherwise there is a perfect groove in the front of your pelvis just below the anterior superior iliac spine where the bar will sit. Your hands are on the bar just outside of your hips to help maintain bar position. The med ball is held between your thighs in an isometric contraction.

Movement

Engage your core, maintain a solid squeeze of the med ball, and engage your glutes to bring your hips off of the floor. Raise your hips to a point where the hip and knee are in line and hold this position for a second, squeezing the glutes.

Finish

After holding the extended position for a second, lower back to the starting position and repeat the rep. Try not to rest on the floor between repetitions.

Tips and Progressions

- Do not allow your lower back to hyperextend.
- If you feel this in the lower back, you are not using your glutes effectively. If this is the case, lower the weight to a manageable load.

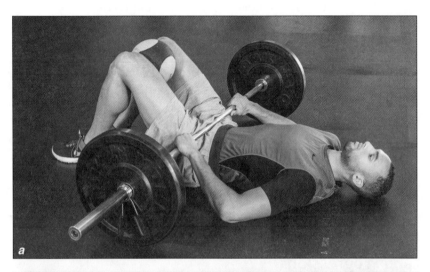

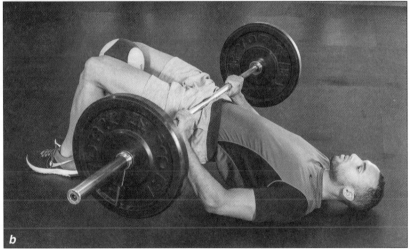

Stability Ball Reverse Rollout

This movement is very similar to the kneeling stability ball rollout detailed in chapter 4. The main difference here is that movement is coming from the opposite end of the body, providing a different mechanical challenge.

Setup

In a power rack, set up the bar at about hip height. Have the stability ball close by; after placing your hands on the bar at shoulder width, kneel on top of the ball.

Movement

Engage your core so you can maintain a neutral spine during the movement. Begin to roll the ball backward until a point where you are just short of full hip extension.

Finish

Once you have reached the end position, keep your abdominals engaged and roll the ball back to the starting position.

Tips and Progressions

If you find the exercise too difficult to start, you can keep your shoulders over the bar and just lengthen your torso as demonstrated in the picture.

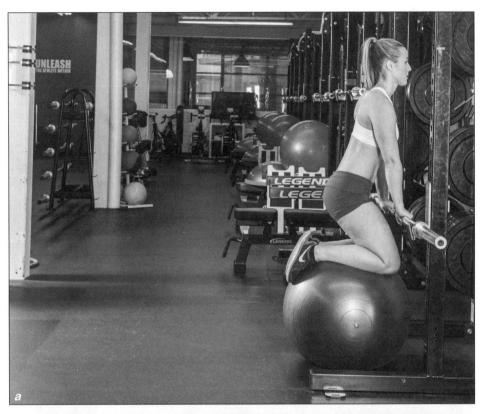

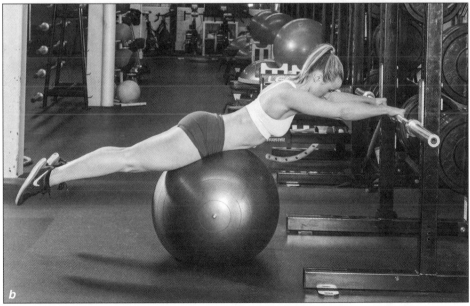

Hanging Knee Raise With Medicine Ball

This classic exercise adds hip compression and load to accentuate the adductors and anterior abdominal sling working together.

Setup

Hang from a bar with an overhand grip, lengthening through the lats, while a partner positions a medicine ball between your knees. Draw the feet up so the knees are in a flexed position.

Movement

Hold the arms static while lifting the knees up to hip height.

Finish

Slowly lower under control back to the setup position.

Tips and Progressions

- Lift the knees up higher, exerting to find any extra range of motion.
- Pausing at the top before lowering more slowly exponentially increases muscle time under tension.
- Introduce more intense recruitment of the adductor muscles by squeezing harder with the legs for isometric strength work here.
- Adding a pull-up magnifies the strength overloading and metabolic cost.

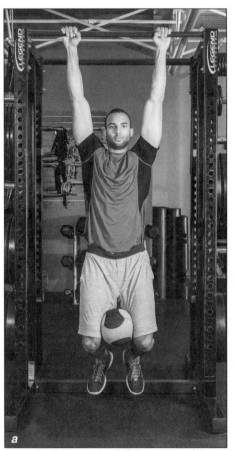 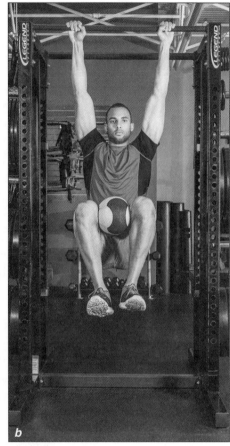

Abdominal Side Crunch

This exercise focuses on the muscles that allow you to bend side to side: the obliques and quadratus lumborum. These muscles are important for flexibility and stability of your core.

Setup

Place a ball approximately three to four feet (about a meter) from a wall. Sit on the ball so that your hips are at the apex of the ball and your feet are against the wall. Stabilize your feet against the wall so you do not roll forward. Lie across the ball so you bend laterally over it.

Movement

From the supported position, begin by crunching laterally until your knees, hips, and shoulders are all in line.

Finish

Once you have reached the position where your body is in line, return to the starting position, ensuring that you fully extend back over the ball.

Tips and Progressions

- As in the abdominal crunch, there are many variations for the side crunch. You can progress from holding your arms across your chest to holding your hands by your ears and then extending your arms over your head.
- You can add an external load by holding a dumbbell in front of your chest.
- By using a medicine ball, you can add a ballistic component to the drill by performing a side crunch throw to a partner.

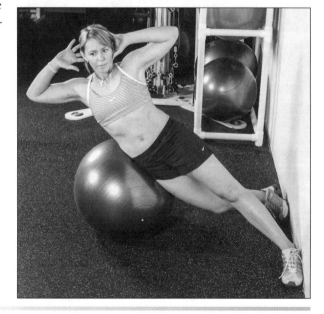

Ball Sit-Up to Medicine Ball Pass

The medicine ball pass adds a dynamic load to a foundational abdominal exercise. Catching a medicine ball imposes distally loaded torque, which must be absorbed and decelerated under control. An additional challenge is the instability at the top of the stability ball where body weight loads and on the floor at the bottom of the stability ball.

Setup

Partner A is positioned on the stability ball, sitting about one-third of the way down the front side of the ball with feet flat on the floor and hip-width apart. With little or no movement of the stability ball, partner A rolls back on the ball, allowing the back to conform around the ball. Partner A has the medicine ball in the hands, ready to do a chest pass to partner B at the end of the sit-up. Partner B stands about four feet (approximately a meter) away from partner A in a good athletic stance, ready to give and receive the medicine ball passes.

Movement

From the start position, partner A engages the abdominal wall and sits up—not curls up—keeping the neck in a neutral position. As partner A approaches the top phase of the sit-up, partner A chest passes the ball to partner B, releasing the ball from the fingertips.

Middle Position

At the top phase, partner A should have the abdominal wall engaged in a neutral alignment from the hips to the neck. The hip joint is angled slightly greater than 90 degrees. In this position the low back is off the ball, and the glutes are on the top, front side of the ball. In the middle position, the core remains contracted. If partner A continues forward to a point at which the core relaxes, lean back slightly until the core engages again. In this position, partner A has the hands out in front, creating the target for partner B to pass the ball back.

Finish

Partner B chest passes the ball back to partner A, who absorbs the pass by immediately engaging the core muscles and rolls back down to the start position.

Tips and Progressions

- Start off with slow, controlled sit-ups and partner passes from chest to chest.
- To advance, increase the weight of the medicine ball, increase the rep count, or increase the tempo of both the throw velocity and sit-up speed.
- Another challenge can be added by increasing the length of partner A's levers by extending the arms overhead during the throw and catch. In this variation, in the down phase of the sit-up, the ball is held overhead instead of in front of the chest.

CHAPTER 10

BICEPS, TRICEPS, AND FOREARMS

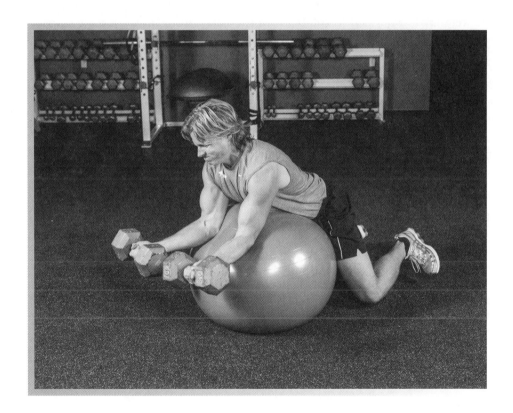

Eccentric Accentuated Biceps Curl

An eccentric contraction occurs when a muscle lengthens under load. Eccentric contractions are known to be significantly stronger than concentric contractions (in which a muscle shortens under load). In the biceps curl movement, as you lower the weight, you can actually lower a heavier weight than what you could raise. If you work on emphasizing the eccentric portion of the movement, your potential concentric (lifting) strength will increase.

Setup

Use a ball that will allow you to lie over it prone with your arms fully extended. Select a weight that is 20 to 40 percent heavier than what you would normally use.

Movement

Since the weight is significantly heavier than what you would normally use, to raise the weight you will need to roll back on the ball. This rolling back will provide you with a mechanical advantage, assisting you in raising the weight.

Finish

Once you have the weight in a fully flexed position, roll back so that your upper arm is back in the downward extended position. Begin by extending your elbow very slowly. It should take you four to six seconds to lower the weight. Once your arm is fully extended, reposition yourself for the next repetition.

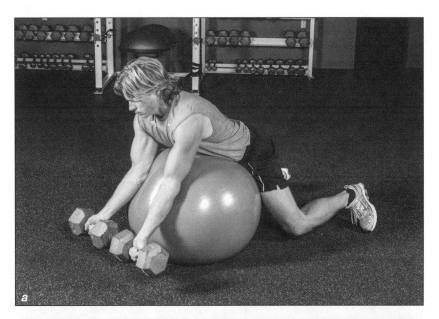

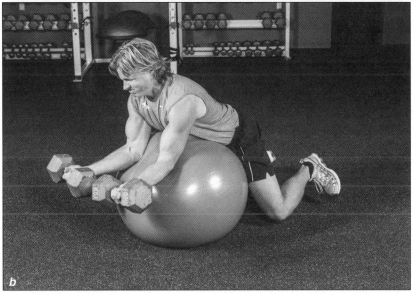

Incline Triceps Extension

The incline triceps extension provides a great challenge to the triceps muscle, specifically the long head of the triceps. As a result of the overhead position of the arms, the long head will get a little more work than the other parts of the triceps.

Setup

Lie over the stability ball on your back. Once in this position, roll forward to a position in which the ball supports your head, shoulders, and back. Once in this position, raise your arms overhead in an extended position with dumbbells in hand.

Movement

While maintaining an erect upper arm, bend at the elbow joint, lowering the dumbbells to a point where you reach full elbow flexion. The dumbbells should be on each side of your head at this point.

Finish

To finish this movement, return to the starting position. Keep your elbows pointing straight up, which will provide optimal isolation for your triceps.

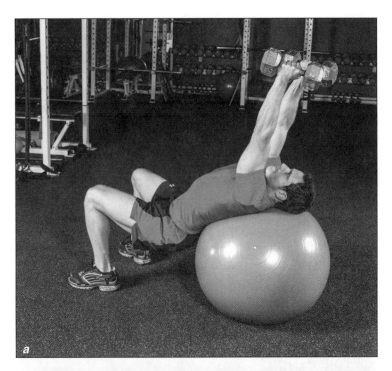

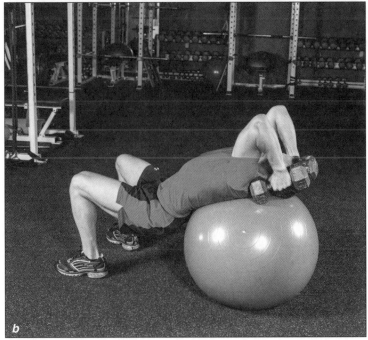

Overhead Medicine Ball Wall Bounce

This drill challenges speed and hand reaction. The movement itself is specific to a throw-in in soccer and overhead pass in basketball. In sports, speed and explosive movement are critical factors, and this movement allows you to move fast.

Setup

Stand approximately 3 to 4 feet (~1 m) away from a wall, with your body in a good athletic position with your core engaged. Hold the medicine ball overhead and flex your elbows so that the ball is actually held behind your head. Elbows should point directly toward the ceiling.

Movement

While you maintain your elbow position, rapidly extend your elbows so that you release the ball toward the wall. Maintain your core position while extending the elbows.

Finish

The ball will come off the wall very quickly. Make sure your hands are ready to accept the ball. The momentum of the ball off the wall will provide a ballistic stretch to your triceps. This elastic loading is then used in reloading and following through on your next rep.

Tips and Progressions

Think of the ball as a hot lava rock. You do not want to hold on to a ball that is hot for very long. The less time you spend with the ball in your hands, the more you will develop the elastic properties of the triceps muscle.

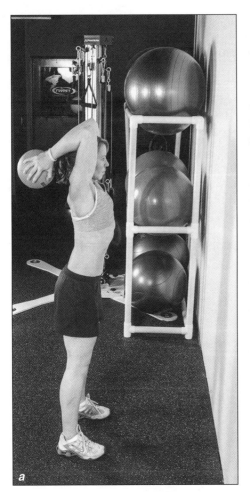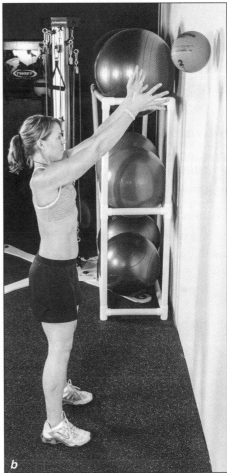

Triceps Blaster

This is an advanced exercise that you should attempt only if you are very experienced. Attempt this first with the feet on the floor; as you become stronger you can perform it with the feet raised on a bench.

Setup

Place both hands on the ball and the feet on the floor with your back in a tight supported position with your abdominals drawn in.

Movement

Holding your back and posture in a very tight position, begin the movement by dropping your elbows toward the floor. The movement can be described as wrapping your forearms down and around the ball.

Finish

As you reach the bottom position after dropping your elbows, your body will be challenged to stay on the ball. Maintain your position and extend your arms to bring yourself back to the starting position.

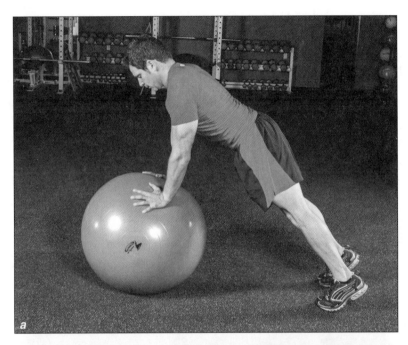

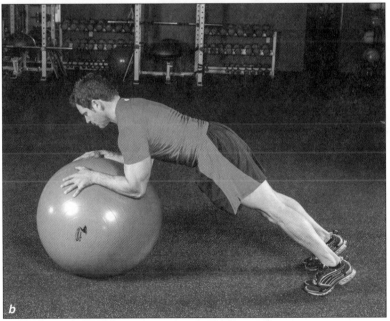

Medicine Ball Push-Up

This exercise uses the simplicity of push-ups and adds balance, core stability, and increased strength requirements.

Setup

Place a medicine ball in front of you. Get into prone position with the hands on the ball in push-up position. Set abdominals to maintain a strong trunk (straight line from ankles to shoulders). Hands are at 3 o'clock and 9 o'clock on the ball. For a greater challenge place feet together to create a small platform, increasing the balance requirements.

Movement

Keeping a rigid core, flex the elbows and lower under control, moving the chest toward the top of the ball.

Finish

Hold and balance before extending the arms to push the body back up in a push-up position.

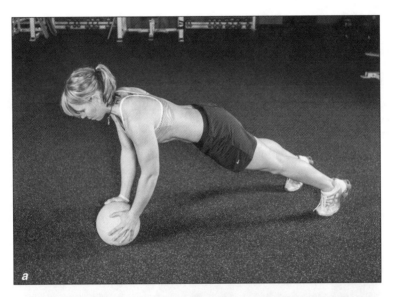

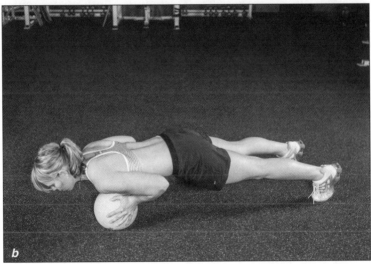

Medicine Ball Walk-Over

Walk-overs are similar to push-ups but activate many more muscles to handle the uneven surfaces and single-arm loading.

Setup

Place a ball in front of you. Get into prone position with the hands on the ball in push-up position. Set the abdominals to maintain a strong trunk (straight line from ankles to shoulders). Remove your left hand and set it on the floor to the left of the ball. Feet remain in place, but upper-body load shifts over to the left arm (floor hand) as you lower onto the left arm.

Movement

Extend the left arm, then push up and over the ball. Transfer your weight onto the right hand as the left hand leaves the floor and joins the right hand on the ball. Once stable, shift your weight onto the left hand and pick up the right hand, placing it on the floor off to the right of the ball.

Finish

Shift your weight over to the right arm. Lower into a push-up position. Continue this sequence until fatigue prevents safe execution.

Tips and Progressions

- Power-over: Using the same general technique and progression, power-overs add a plyometric action.
- When extending the floor (left) arm, powerfully drive up to propel the torso into the air.
- The right hand leaves the ball slightly before the left hand lands on the ball.
- The torso shifts left and right with speed.
- When the right hand reaches the floor, quickly flex the elbow to drop into a push-up position and immediately explode back up, pushing the torso back up and over the ball.
- The hands dance back and forth, executing this drill with speed.

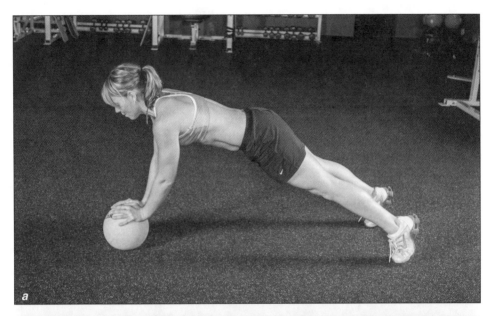

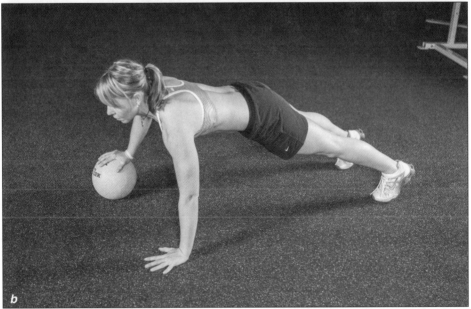

Wrist Curl and Extension

The setup is the same for both wrist curls and wrist extensions. Flexion and extension of the wrist are areas that traditionally have been ignored in strengthening programs, mainly because people think that these muscles receive enough work during other gripping exercises.

Setup

Set up in front of an adjustable cable column, or hold dumbbells, as shown in the photos. Set the column so that the pulley is approximately 20 degrees below the top of the ball.

Movement

Grasping the bar with an underhand grip for the curl movement, begin in the fully extended position and flex your wrists through a full range of motion. Hold this position for a second or two.

Finish

Slowly lower the weight back to the original position. Note: For the extension movement, palms begin facing the floor.

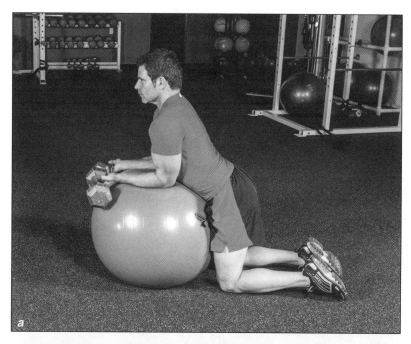

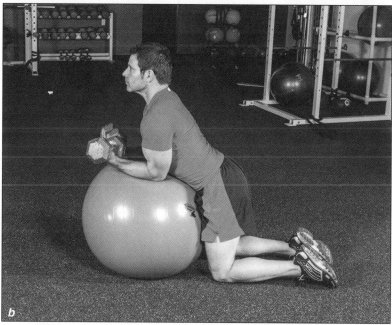

Medicine Ball Quick Drop and Catch

Grip strength and forearm development are important for sports that require grip on an implement or object. Holding on to a hockey stick or tennis racket and a pump fake in football are examples of the need for grip strength with integrated forearm movement.

Setup

Begin in an athletic position facing your partner, who is holding a smaller-diameter medicine ball. Place your hands in a pronated, or palms-down, position. Your elbows should be in close to your body at 90-degree angles.

Movement

The exercise begins when your partner releases the ball. After the release, very quickly extend your elbows eccentrically in the direction of the dropping ball.

Finish

Catch the ball within 4 to 6 inches (10 to 15 cm) of its drop, and flex the elbows back up so that you have 90-degree angles at the elbows.

Tips and Progressions

- This movement should be completed very fast.
- Think of the ball as being very hot. If you hold on too long, you will burn your hand.

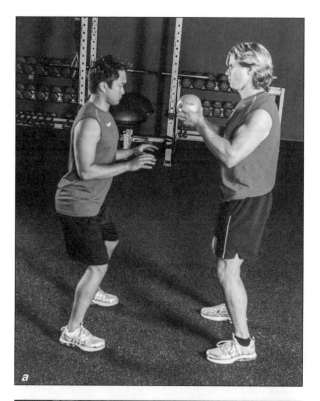

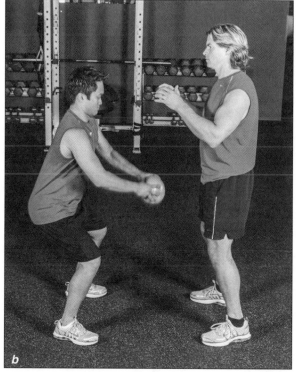

CHAPTER 11

WHOLE BODY

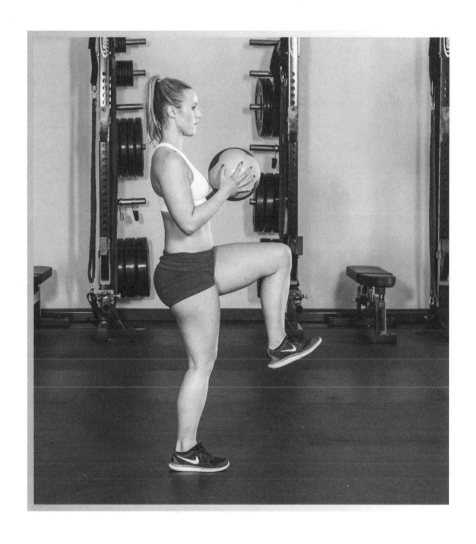

Medicine Ball Squat-Away

Using two primal moves, the body must move into a very low deep position before it rises up to its longest length. Shortening and lengthening muscles crossing joints while using the joints functionally across their widest capability improves freedom of motion through the kinetic chain.

Setup

Adjust your foot placement into a wide athletic-ready position with the stability ball held in front of you close to the body in a row position.

Movement

Squat as deep as possible, aiming to drop your hips below knee height. Be careful to keep your torso as upright as possible and your shoulders back. As you squat down, move the ball away from the body, pressing it out in front of the body, arms extended. Find as much length there as possible.

Finish

Stand up as you pull the ball back in tight to your torso, initiating the pull with your back and not the arms.

Tips and Progressions

- Change the base of support by widening or narrowing the foot stance.
- Take extra time at the very bottom and top to permit the body the time it needs to ease into greater ranges of motion.
- Once mobility improves, close your eyes to layer a light proprioceptive over-load and train internal body awareness through those fluid ranges of ability.

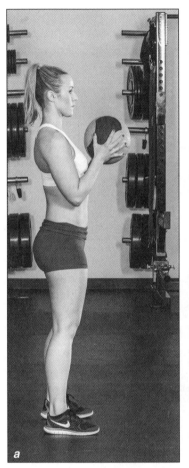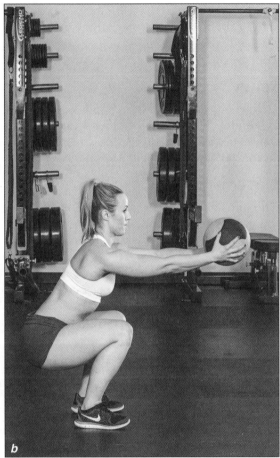

Prone Stability Ball Three-Way Hip Drill

Building core strength in the unstable prone hold position, you move the foot and leg about to integrate with three primary hip actions showing mobility around a braced core. These three actions are a knee tuck, a straight-leg hip raise, and a deep forward lunge.

Setup

Assume a push-up position, hands on the stability ball, chest over the ball, and toes on the floor about shoulder-width apart. Use a hand placement that is most comfortable for you; often, this is accomplished by placing the heel of the hands on the top side of the ball, with the fingers wrapped over the sides of the ball.

Movement

One side at a time, pick up the foot to bring the knee in tight to the chest, then straighten the leg completely as you kick the heel toward the ceiling.

Finish

Complete the rep by stepping into a lunge, bringing the foot to land outside the ball parallel to the hand placement. This unloads the arms and hands and stretches down the low back around the glutes into the hamstring. Finish tall, keeping hips low and torso upright. Finally, pick up the foot to return to setup position.

Tips and Progression

- Focus and exert to secure longer range of motion in all positions: knee in, leg straight, heel high, lunge.
- Accentuate stability around new mobility by pausing briefly in each of the three positions. This allows more time to strive for added range and forces the muscles to stabilize the three-point stance with those mechanics.

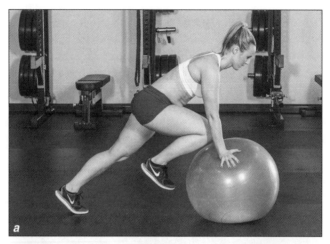

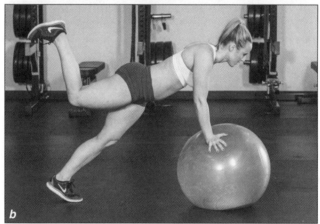

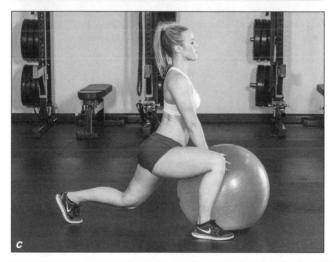

Rollover Agility

David Weck is the creator of the BOSU device and most recently the DSL stability ball. David has created some outstanding exercises with the BOSU and the DSL ball. This is just one of his exercises that combines functional agility with a fun movement. The ball allows you to complete rolling movements safely without the impact usually associated with this type of athletic drill.

Setup

Get in position beside the ball in a deep split stance with the outside leg forward and inside hand on the floor.

Movement

Drop the torso onto the ball and roll right over, exiting off the opposite side.

Finish

Land in a deep split with the outside leg forward and inside hand on the floor to help steady the body. Finish with your head up, visually aware, before returning across the ball to the first side.

Tips and Progressions

- Begin slowly, striving for control and consistency.
- When you become proficient, start to increase the tempo.

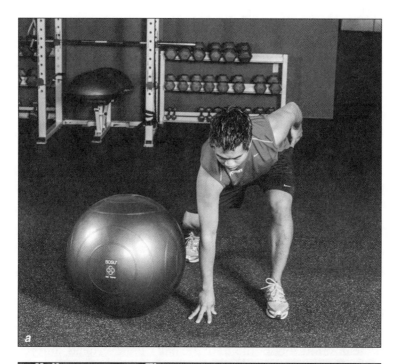

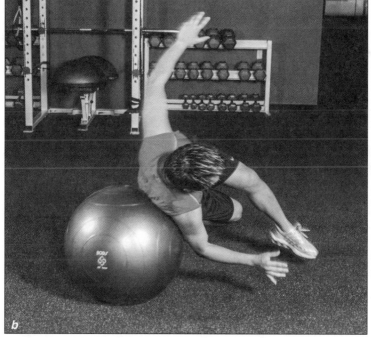

Walking Lunge With Overhead Medicine Ball Rotation

The walking lunge on its own is quite a challenging exercise. When you add the load of the medicine ball with overhead rotation, you create a movement that encompasses flexion, extension, and rotation. Although the prime mover is the legs, this movement challenges the whole body.

Setup

Begin in a split position so that the front of the tibia is perpendicular to the floor with a 90-degree angle at the knee. If you begin with your left leg in front, you will hold the ball with the core rotated to the left and the ball on the outside of the left hip.

Movement

To initiate movement, press the left foot into the floor, which will initiate extension of the left hip and left quad. As this firing of the quad and hip begins, raise the ball in a half-circle motion overhead. The right leg also begins to step forward with the goal of becoming the forward plant leg.

Middle Position

In the middle position you should have the ball right overhead, and your left leg should be fully extended.

Finish

As the right foot comes forward and lowers into a flexed position at the knee, the ball continues to move overhead in the half-circle motion to finish on the opposite hip.

Tips and Progressions

You can also use this walking lunge movement with a static overhead medicine ball hold. This provides greater challenge to the posterior chain musculature, which promotes proper posture.

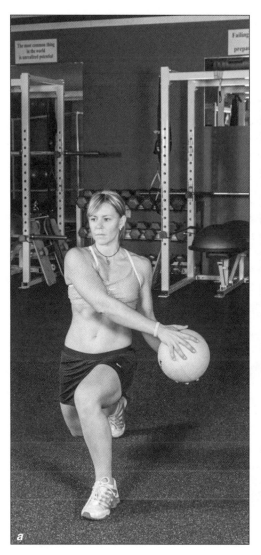 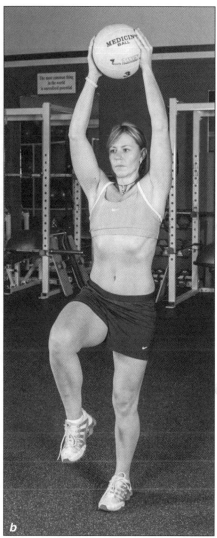

Angle Lunge With Horizontal Medicine Ball Rotation

This exercise is similar to the walking lunge. The difference is that this is performed while in place, with a greater challenge to the medial adductors of the thigh.

Setup

Begin in a split position so that the front of the tibia is perpendicular to the floor with a 90-degree angle at the knee and the hip abducted to approximately 30 to 40 degrees. If you begin with your left leg in front, the ball will be held with the core rotated to the left and arms extended straight out at chest height.

Movement

To initiate movement, press the left foot into the floor, which will initiate extension of the left hip and left quad. As this firing of the quad and hip begins, rotate the medicine ball across your body, horizontal to the floor.

Middle Position

In the middle position you should have the ball right in front of your chest and your left leg coming back to the midline of the body. Here is an instantaneous transfer of weight, and the right leg begins to explode to a 30- to 40-degree angle to the right side.

Finish

As the right foot comes forward and lowers into a flexed position at the knee, the ball continues to move across the body to finish on the right side.

Tips and Progressions

If you have difficulty keeping your posture correct as you rotate and move, try shortening the lever by holding the ball closer to the body, and progress to fully extended arms.

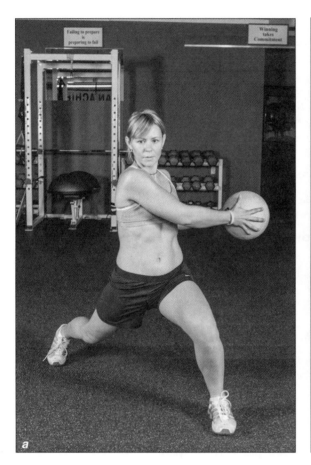

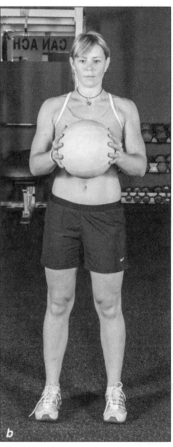

Static Split Lunge to Dumbbell Lateral Raise

This integrated whole-body exercise combines all five pillars of functional performance: strength, stability, mobility, balance, and movement skill. Thus this exercise draws on neural organization and transfers to life and sport.

Setup

Hold a dumbbell close across the body at the opposite hip. Standing tall, place the rear foot atop a stability ball.

Movement

Push the leg back to roll into a long, deep lunge position, raising the dumbbell up laterally.

Finish

Finish with the elbow level with the shoulder, torso level and tall, hips low.

Tips and Progressions

- Increase the strength demands by slowing your tempo of both the body and the arm.
- Add pauses at the peak shoulder movement. Focus on holding the shoulder strong without allowing the torso to deviate.

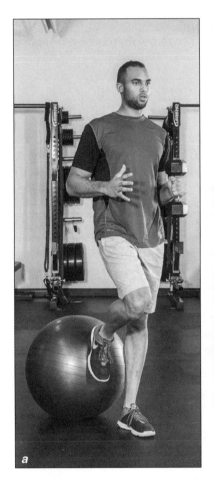 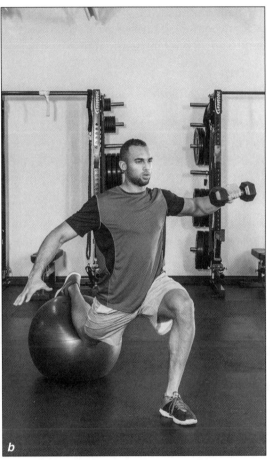

Medicine Ball Romanian Deadlift to Overhead Extension

In many instances in this book we emphasize the importance of training the posterior chain. This is a great whole-body exercise that will help you integrate it into an all-encompassing move.

Setup

Stand in an athletic posture, holding a medicine ball with extended arms.

Movement

Begin the movement by engaging the core and pushing your hips backward while shifting your weight to your heels and not allowing your knees to bend any farther from the original athletic posture. Lower yourself to a point where you can maintain proper low back posture.

Finish

Once you have reached your low position of the Romanian deadlift, come back up toward the starting position but raise the ball with extended arms all the way over your head. Lower the ball back to the starting position and repeat.

Tips and Progressions

Do not allow your low back to flex forward or your knees to flex. In the overhead position reach as high as you can.

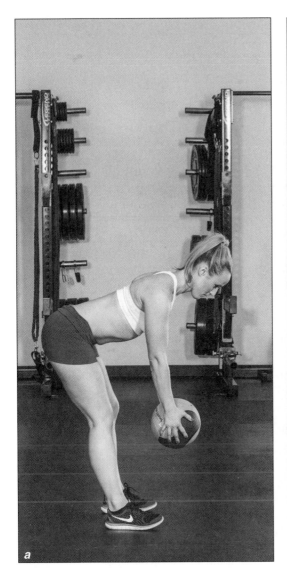
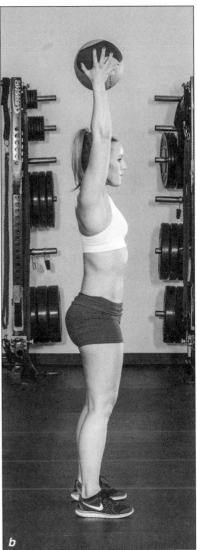

Medicine Ball Romanian Deadlift to Hip Flexion

Where the previous exercise focuses completely on the posterior chain, this one focuses on the extensors on one side and the flexors on the other. The intensity and balance requirement is higher as a result of the single-leg stance.

Setup

In an athletic posture, hold a medicine ball with extended arms and balance on one leg.

Movement

Begin the movement by engaging the core and pushing your hip backward and not allowing your knee to bend any farther from the original athletic posture. Movement must come from the hips. Lower yourself to a point where you can maintain proper low back posture.

Finish

As you begin to rise back up, at the very same time your opposite leg comes up to a hip-flexed position. Once at the top, repeat for the recommended number of reps, then repeat on the opposite side.

Tips and Progressions

- It should look as if your legs are synchronized.
- Never allow your low back to flex forward at the bottom or at the top as you bring your hip up and forward.
- As you become proficient in this movement, you can increase the intensity by switching to a heavier dumbbell.

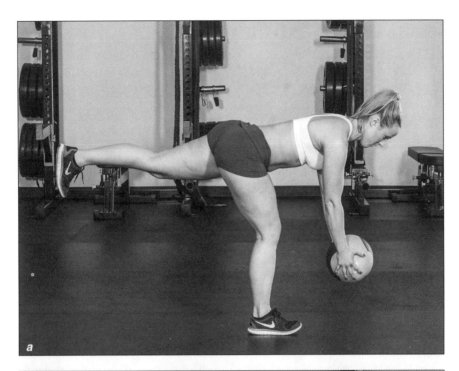

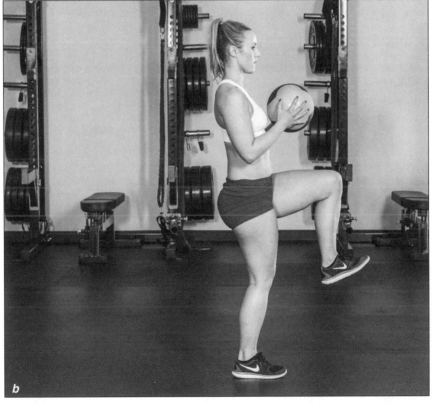

Squat to Ballast Ball to Romanian Deadlift

This movement combines the fundamental benefits of the squat with the Romanian deadlift.

Setup

Stand in an athletic posture holding a medicine ball behind your head or dumbbells by your sides with extended arms.

Movement

Initiate by engaging your core with your chest up and shoulders depressed to fully lock in your spine. Squat onto the ballast ball but do not rest there; keep all muscles engaged.

Finish

After pausing for a second, rise up out of the squat, keep your feet in the same position, then begin the Romanian deadlift movement by pushing your hips backward, all the while shifting your weight to your heels and not allowing your knees to bend any farther from the original athletic posture. Lower yourself to a point where you can maintain proper low back posture, and return.

Tips and Progressions

- As you transition from one movement to the other, make sure you maintain your core stability.
- When squatting, do not allow your upper body to flex forward. The focus should be on your hips, knees, and ankles.

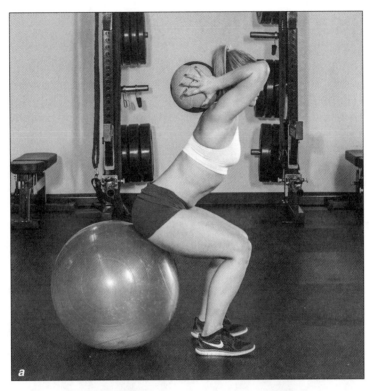

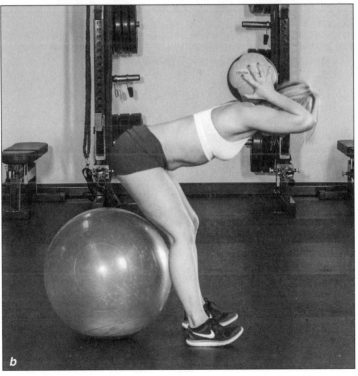

Ax Chop With Hip Flexion

This movement ties in the functional line of the right external oblique, left hip adductor, psoas, and rectus femoris. This line of pull can be traced from the top of the right ilium to the middle outer thigh. These muscles all function together to provide rotation to the left. The movement should begin with a moderate pace.

Setup

Get in a solid athletic stance with your feet approximately shoulder-width apart. Holding the ball with both hands, flex your arms up so that the ball is up over the shoulder. Slide your opposite leg back on an angle of approximately 30 degrees.

Movement

Begin the movement by simultaneously chopping down with the ball and flexing your opposite hip up with a slight adduction. This will produce a crisscross of the ball and your upper thigh.

Finish

Once the ball has met the outside of the thigh, reverse the movement quickly and return to the start position.

Tips and Progressions

- Once you feel comfortable with a moderate speed, progress to a more explosive movement.
- You can provide added resistance to the hip flexors and adductors by attaching rubber tubing or a cable to your ankle.

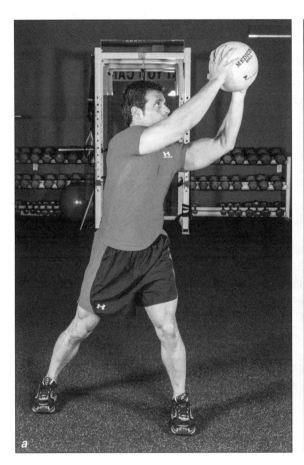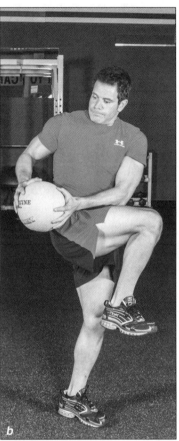

Medicine Ball Overhead Lateral Bounce to Floor

This drill requires some coordination in driving the ball into the floor at the correct angle to catch and reverse the movement.

Setup

With feet shoulder-width apart, raise the ball overhead and over to one side. Set your core and prepare to drive the ball downward.

Movement

Success in this drill is determined by the angle needed to receive the ball. As you drive the ball down from your outside shoulder, you want to hit a midpoint on the floor between your feet. This will cause the ball to bounce up on an angle toward the opposite shoulder.

Finish

Once you have released the ball, your arms move to the opposite side to meet the ball and begin deceleration. The bounce of the ball should take your hands up to the opposite shoulder. Then explode the ball back in the opposite direction.

Tips and Progressions

Begin this movement with a lighter ball in the 6- to 8-pound range (~2.5 to 3.5 kg), and slowly progress until you can handle a 12- to 15-pound (~ 5.5 to 6.5 kg) medicine ball.

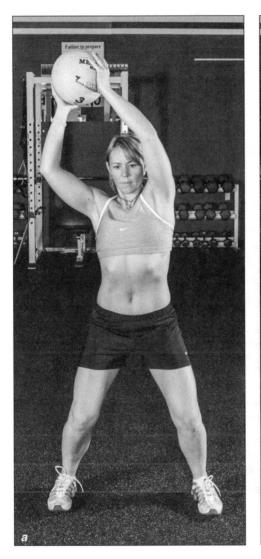
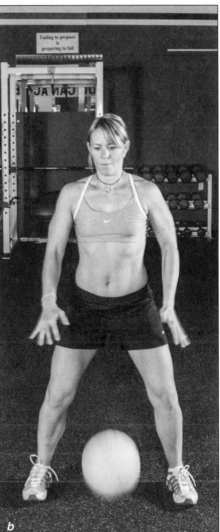

Medicine Ball Overhead Jump and Throw

This exercise may very well be the most integrated explosive medicine ball exercise you can perform. It requires an explosive triple extension of the body (integration of the ankles, knees, and hips). This movement is important if you play football, compete in track and field events, or would just like to work on your total-body explosiveness.

Setup

With feet shoulder-width apart and your body in a set athletic position, hold the medicine ball so it hangs right below your shoulders at approximately knee level.

Movement

Begin the movement by driving your hips forward and pressing your feet into the floor. This will be a powerful and fast muscle contraction. This initial drive results in a force in which your body propels itself upward in a jumping motion.

Finish

As your body drives upward, integrate the upward movement of the ball. Use the momentum of your jump and transfer that force to the ball. Release the ball as your arms rise to the highest point of your jump.

Tips and Progressions

- Begin this movement with a lighter ball in the 12- to 15-pound range (~5.5 to 6.5 kg), and slowly progress until you can handle a 25- to 30-pound (~11 to 13.5 kg) medicine ball. This heavier weight will challenge your nervous system.

- You can drive the ball either straight up into the air or in a backward arc. When the ball goes straight up, make sure you do not try to catch it. Get out of the way and let it fall to the floor. When throwing back in an arc, you should be outdoors and ensure no one is in the ball's path.

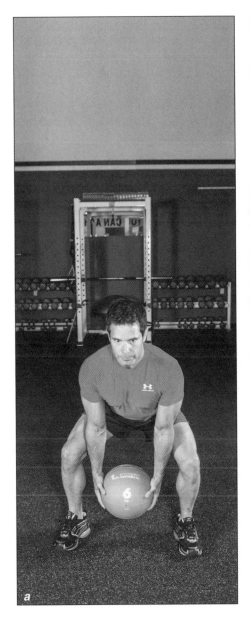 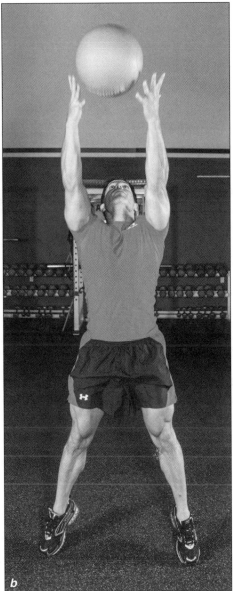

Medicine Ball Throw Two-Leg Jump to Single-Leg Lateral Land

This drill is excellent for coordination and power combined. It involves power in both the sagittal and frontal planes and deceleration, which are important for sports that require changes in direction.

Setup

You should be approximately 8 to 10 feet (2.4 to 3 m) from a solid wall or a partner that you can throw the ball into. Be set in an athletic stance while holding the ball close to the chest at chest height.

Movement

This movement is quite complex and you may want to refer to the video clip that demonstrates the technique for this exercise. The initial movement involves simultaneously driving the ball into the wall and jumping forward.

Finish

As you propel yourself forward, you must turn 90 degrees and land on your inside leg closest to the wall. Stabilize when you land, and catch the ball as it comes off the wall. Once you catch the ball, reset your position and repeat.

Tips and Progressions

You can try progressing your single-leg landing to the outside leg, which will stress the landing adductors. Before attempting with the ball, try a few repetitions without the ball and make sure you are familiar with the footwork.

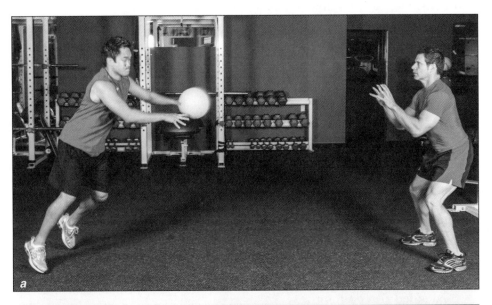

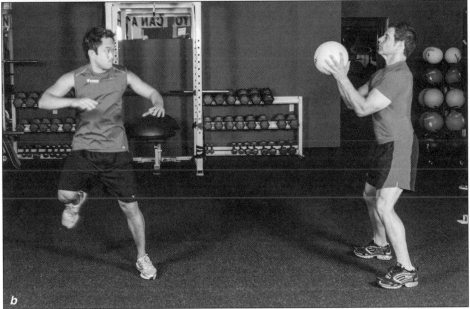

Medicine Ball Circuit

This minicircuit is a combination of four movements in one giant set. It will tax your core as well as your anaerobic energy system.

Overhead Chop

- Set up in a solid athletic stance, feet shoulder-width apart, with your chest and shoulders just over your knees. Hold a medicine ball with your arms fully extended so that the ball is between your knees. Set your core before initiating the following movement.
- Swing your arms straight up hard so the ball will move up overhead, just as you might swing an ax (see figure *a*).
- Once you have reached the overhead position, reverse your movement as fast as you can, and drive the ball back down with a powerful chop. Reverse the movement again and continue until you complete 10 chops.
- Once you have completed the 10 overhead chops, the second consecutive movement is the overhead lateral side bend.

Overhead Lateral Side Bend

- Maintaining the same athletic stance, hold the ball overhead in a fully extended arm position.
- Set your core and laterally flex at your waist so you bend over to one side (see figure *b*). Do not allow any lateral movement as you flex sideways.
- Once you have flexed laterally as far as you can, reverse the direction to the opposite side. The movement speed should not be explosive, but it should be fast. Complete 10 flexions to each side, then move on to the standing twist.

Standing Twist

- Continue the same solid athletic stance, and flex your arms forward so the ball is held out front at chest level.
- Using an explosive movement, rotate to one side. Ensure that you follow the ball with your eyes and head as you turn (see figure *c*).
- Once you have reached your full range of rotation, explosively rotate back to the opposite side, again following the ball with your eyes and head. Complete 10 rotations to each side.
- The final exercise is the ax chop with hip flexion, which ties in the upper and lower body in a complex movement.

Ax Chop With Hip Flexion

- Immediately after your last standing rotation, move the ball up over one shoulder, and slide the opposite leg back on an angle of approximately 30 degrees.
- Begin the movement by simultaneously chopping down with the ball and flexing your opposite hip up with a very fast movement (see figure *d*).

- Once the ball has met the outside of the thigh, return to the original start position. Complete 10 repetitions to each side and then rest.
- Once you have completed one full minicircuit, rest 60 to 120 seconds and repeat three or four circuits.

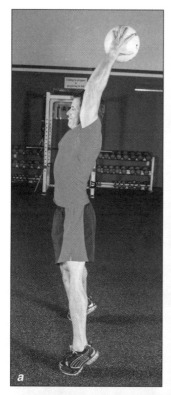
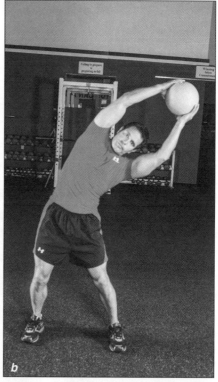

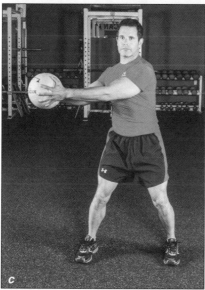
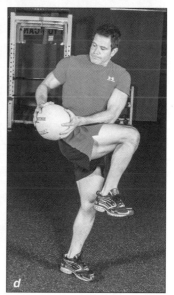

CHAPTER 12

FLEXIBILITY

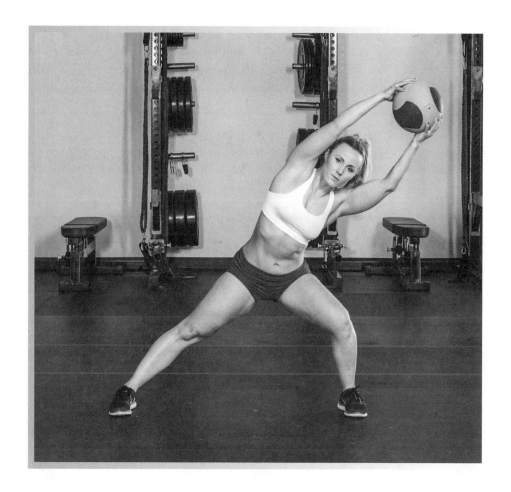

Spinal Extension

Mobility in the spine is essential if the rest of the body is to function efficiently. As with strengthening, stretching the spine in multiple planes and angles will assist in spinal health. The spinal extension is a safe method of placing a stretch on the anterior ligaments and muscles of the spinal column as well as the abdominals.

Setup

Sitting on a ball, walk forward until the ball lies in the natural curve of your lower back.

Movement

Rock forward and backward by pressing your legs into the floor. This will force the ball to roll back. Follow the roll of the ball, which will provide the stretch to the abdominals. The farther you roll back, the greater the stretch. Begin with smaller rolls at first and then progress to larger rolls.

Finish

Once you have reached your end range, hold the stretch for 8 to 15 seconds, and then return. This stretch time is shorter than for most stretches because with your head in this position, you may feel slightly dizzy if you stay in the stretched position for an extended period.

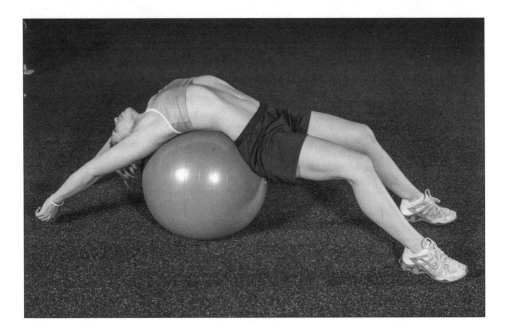

Lateral Side Stretch

This drill provides a stretch for the all-important side-flexing spinal muscles as well as the obliques.

Setup

Place a ball approximately three to four feet (about a meter) from a wall. Sit on the ball so that your hips are at the apex of the ball and your feet are against the wall. Stabilize your feet against the wall so you do not roll forward. Lie across the ball so you bend laterally over it.

Movement

There is no movement once you have reached the stretched position.

Finish

Hold the stretched position over the ball for 20 to 30 seconds, then repeat on the opposite side.

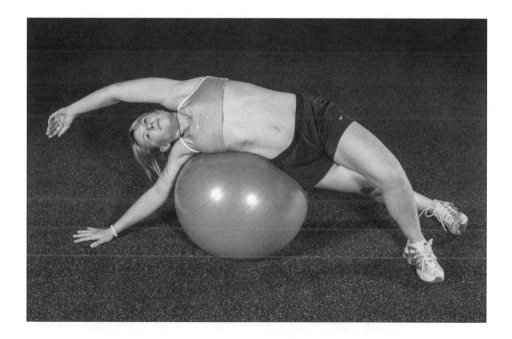

Standing Hamstring Stretch

Stretching the hamstring from the standing position will emphasize the upper part of the muscle toward the hip.

Setup

Place your foot on top of a ball.

Movement

Maintain your lordotic curve in the lower back, and slowly flex forward. Focus on moving your navel toward your thigh. At the same time as you flex forward, press your heel gently into the ball. Hold this contraction for five to six seconds, relax the stretch for two seconds, and then proceed into the next stretch. This uses the proprioceptive neuromuscular facilitation (PNF) method of stretching, which means that if you contract a muscle, allow it to relax, and then stretch it again, the subsequent stretch will be greater. You can also focus on the different heads of the hamstrings by pointing your toes in and out.

Finish

Perform three to five static stretches of 20 to 30 seconds, or two or three sets of three or four PNF stretches.

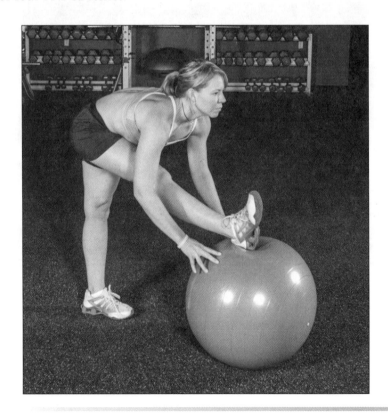

Kneeling Posterior Shoulder Stretch

Stretching the posterior side of the shoulder is important for mobility and complete range of motion at the shoulder joint.

Setup

Kneel in front of a ball, with the ball slightly off to the left side. Move your right arm across your body and place it on the ball.

Movement

Begin to roll the ball to the left by pushing with the right hand. As you reach the end of the range, flex forward. This places a greater stretch on the posterior fibers of the deltoid and the rhomboid, which spans the space between your shoulder blade and your upper spine.

Finish

Hold the stretch for 20 to 30 seconds and return to the initial position. Repeat three to five times.

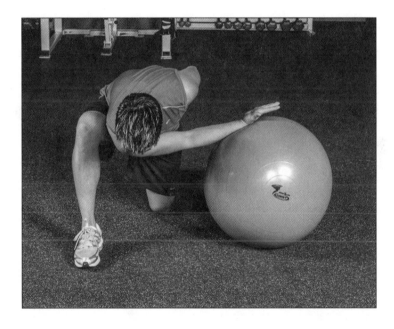

Stability Ball Thoracic Mobility

Thoracic mobility is one of the key aspects of a healthy spine. As a rotational movement, this exercise allows you to assess your progression in range of motion and compare your level of strength on your left and right sides.

Setup

With your knees hip-width apart, kneel on the floor in front of a stability ball. Roll the ball forward by extending your hips so your body is in a tabletop position with your arms resting over the ball.

Movement

Begin the movement by rotating to one side, turning the ball with your body. Your head, neck, and spine should move as one unit. Do not lose your lower lumbar positioning.

Finish

Once you have you reached the end of the range of motion, reverse the movement to rotate to the other side.

Tips and Progressions

- The key to success in this exercise is the body moving as a single unit.
- Do not allow your lower back to dip as you move through the range of motion.
- Turn your eyes up toward the high elbow to increase the challenge.

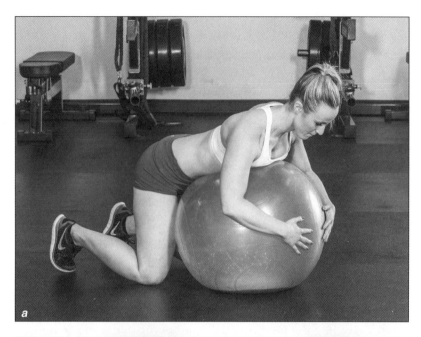

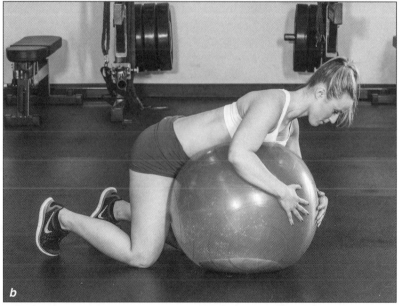

Rainbow Squat

Setup

Holding a medicine ball, assume a very wide parallel foot placement.

Movement

Shift the hips over laterally to one side and reach the medicine ball outside the body to the same side, avoiding lateral torso flexion.

Finish

Bring the medicine ball from wide outside the body to high overhead in an arced rainbow pattern. As hips shift over to load the other leg, bring the ball all the way over and across to that side.

Tips and Progressions

- As range of motion opens up, reestablish a new setup position with wider foot stance.
- Focus on shifting the hips so the hips lead, avoiding the tendency to break at the hips with the side bending into the medicine ball movement.
- When beginning the medicine ball rainbow up and over the body, initiate the pull at the hips and feel muscle movement up the side of your torso to lead that action.

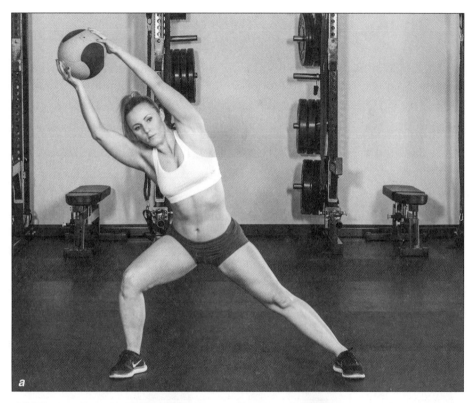

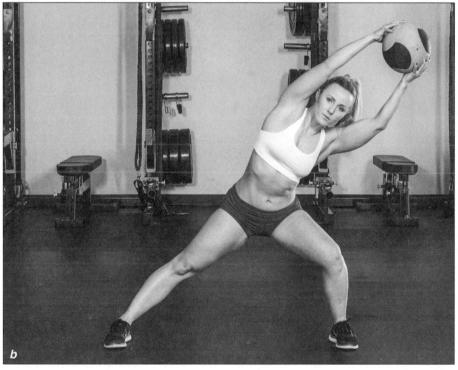

Standing Lat and Pec Stretch

The latissimus dorsi and pectorals are two muscle groups that, if not stretched effectively, can restrict range of motion in the shoulder. Flexibility in this area is essential for overall shoulder health, especially for throwing athletes.

Setup

Take a split stance with your left foot forward. Place a ball between your right hand and the wall.

Movement

Begin by rolling the ball straight up the wall until the arm is fully extended. To increase the stretch on the shoulder, lunge forward slightly. Hold the stretch position for 20 to 30 seconds, and return to the original position. You can also perform this dynamically by increasing the speed of the ball roll and lunge.

Finish

Perform three to five static stretches of 20 to 30 seconds or two or three sets of 10 dynamic stretches.

CHAPTER 13

STRENGTH BALL PROGRAMS

Since the release of the second edition of this book, we have had some incredible feedback on the initial programs. The third edition contains targeted programs that meet specific needs. So no matter your goal or your clients' goals, you will hit the mark. If you want to gain some muscle mass, then you have to check out the muscle up program. Has an injury been setting you back, or are you are looking to start training again? Then the body reset will help you get functional and moving again. Eight new programs focus on all the hottest developments in the market—but they're backed up by science.

Remember you can still go back to the 16-week program. It remains in this edition if you are new to strength ball training. If have already completed the 16-week program, it's time to ramp it up with more load or repetitions or both to challenge yourself to the max.

Warm-Up and Movement Preparation

Jumping into your workout without a proper warm-up would not be beneficial to your body. You might be able to relate it to starting your car and immediately trying to drive it on a freezing February morning in Ottawa. You must first start it and then let it warm up so the oil can work its way around the moving engine parts. Your body is no different. Begin by slowly raising your body temperature with 5 to 8 minutes of aerobic activity. Then perform some dynamic activity to lubricate your joints, such as walking lunges, rotating lunges, hip swings, medicine ball ax chops, or robot arms.

Rationale for Program Development

When we design exercise programs for our clients, we take several factors into consideration:

1. The sport the athlete is preparing for

2. Training goals, such as reducing body fat, increasing strength, or increasing muscle mass

3. Chronological age

4. Training age (number of years of resistance and balance training a client has)

5. Injury history

6. Sex

7. Equipment availability (whether or not there is access to the appropriate equipment)

The unfortunate part of designing a program for this book is that we cannot get too specific. The design and progressions are carefully planned to provide you with guidelines that will educate you as well as improve your strength. Following are the guidelines that you should use when designing your own program.

Stability and balance are addressed from a physiological perspective in chapters 1 and 2. From a programming perspective, stability and balance are characteristics that we prefer to work on early on in our program design. This does not mean we don't do any balance later in the program; rather, the focus might be different. For instance, early on we might focus on unstable balance with a minor strength component, such as the bridge T fall-off in weeks 1 to 4. This exercise allows you to challenge your balance progressively (that is, you dictate your own balance difficulty by how far you laterally roll with the ball). The more you adapt, the farther you will roll. Once you have reached your maximum lateral roll, you could decrease your base of support, which will increase the balance challenge of just being on top of the ball. Bridge Ts are a great introductory balance exercise because you can dictate your difficulty.

The ability to balance in a three-point stance in the Ts will lend itself positively to balance challenges later in the program when there is only a two-point balance, such as the single-leg hip extension and knee flexion. Not only do you have a two-point balance point, but there is also a significant strength requirement during this balance challenge.

The progressions will dictate future success with your program. Without appropriate progressions, results might not occur. Imagine, for instance, you are just starting out with your strength ball program, and you have programmed in the single-leg hip extension and knee flexion in your first cycle. Most people cannot perform this exercise effectively because they do not have the required balance or stability. In many cases this failure could result in your quitting the program. Fitness dropout rates are common among people who try to do too much too soon and are turned off by the inability to complete a workout.

When we look at the strength component of programming, the thought processes are very similar to that of balance and stability: Build a base and use reasonable progressions. For instance, you would not want to use the dual-ball fly to work your chest at the beginning of your program. This exercise places great stress on the anterior shoulder. It also requires great core stability as you descend into your fly. You will notice that we begin the chest progression by using a bilateral stability ball dumbbell press. This is a great introductory general strength exercise for the pectorals and basic stability exercise for the core. Progress to a unilateral stability ball dumbbell press. This will force the core to work at a much higher level as a result of the unilateral arm movement. After following these progressions for 8 weeks, you might be ready to attempt the dual-ball fly. If you cannot descend in a slow, controlled manner while holding your core in the proper position and rise from the low position, you will know that you are not ready for this progression. If that is the case, take a positive step back to reinforce the muscles that will help you achieve success in the movement.

Stability and Balance (Injury Prevention)

Program Description

Your stability and balance workout uses instability applied overhead from the top down, lever loaded through the arms, and from the ground up through the feet. The exercises demand advanced software computations that increase the muscle activity across joints. The timing and strength of muscle stiffness across joints are important to all tasks, such as walking down stairs. With each foot plant the knees and hips require the right amount of muscle activity at the right time to stabilize each joint and help balance the entire body over the leg that loads. Whole-body balance and joint stability are key to gait patterns and whole-body physical activity. Improving them helps the body be ready to manage advanced exercise challenges like strength and power. Instability and poor balance are common causes of injury.

Complete each exercise twice before progressing to the next exercise. Rest for 30 to 60 seconds between exercises.

Exercise

Bridge ball hold: 2 × 15 rapid

Standing overhead medicine ball rotation: 2 × 10 each way controlled tempo

Prone medicine ball transfer: 2 × 10 each side slow

Ball walk-around: 2 × 3 each way (6 reps total) controlled

Single-leg stride squat: 2 × 12 per leg controlled

Supine push and drive: 2 × 8 per side controlled with pause hold

Stability ball single-leg split squat with dumbbell: 2 × 12 each side slow

Dual-ball survival rollout: 2 × 12 slow with pause

Freedom of Motion (Mobility and Movement Skills)

Program Description

The freedom of motion workout builds flexibility in motion, which translates as mobility, the range of joint motion. Easier and more fluid motion across hip and shoulder joints greatly affect comfort and efficiency in functional movement.

Begin with the first exercise using a controlled or slow tempo (as indicated), concentrating on precise mechanics. Focus effort on finding additional range of motion in each movement. Complete the first exercise and then advance to the next exercise in the workout with as much or as little rest as you need in order to execute the subsequent exercise well.

While you will use strength and stability and effort to accomplish these exercises, the primary goals are skilled movement and mobility, so being more rested and less fatigued works in your favor.

Exercise

Ax chop with hip flexion: 2 × 15 slow

Reverse lunge and rotate: 2 × 8 per side slow

Rainbow squat: 2 × 10 side to side slow

Alternating open-step medicine ball lunge with long lever rotation: 2 × 8 per side slow

Medicine ball squat-away posterior wall chain hold: 2 × 8 per side controlled

Single-leg rotations: 2 × 6 per leg controlled

Walking lunge with overhead medicine ball rotation: 2 × 12 per leg controlled

Prone stability ball three-way hip drill: 2 × 6 controlled

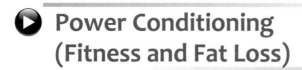

Power Conditioning
(Fitness and Fat Loss)

Program Description

The power conditioning workout harnesses explosive power with exercises of high metabolic cost to burn maximum calories and elevate fitness.

The workout involves four supersets each consisting of two exercises. Complete the first superset (two exercises) without rest before resting for 30 seconds, then move on to the next superset. Rest no more than 30 seconds between each superset.

Finish all four supersets before proceeding through the medicine ball circuit once. Rest a full 2 minutes, drink water, then get ready to do the entire workout two more times through from beginning to end. As fitness develops, extend the rep count per set or add a fourth round of the entire workout.

Exercise

Lunge with medicine ball pass: 3 × 10 passes in each leg position

+ Walk-out to push-up: 3 × 8 reps

Repeated dual-foot long jump: 3 × 12 jumps

+ Up up, down down: 3 × 20 reps (20 times up and down)

Plyometric medicine ball box jump: 3 × 12 jumps

+ Supine stability ball medicine ball chest push to self-catch: 3 × 20 catches

Lateral-jump ball hold: 3 × 8 per side

+ Side-to-side rotation pass: 3 × 8 per side

Medicine ball circuit: 3 times

Abs and Ass (Alternatively named Abs and Butt or Core and Glutes)

Program Description

Exercising the abs and butt is best accomplished using both old-school and new-school principles. Old-school ways of isolating an exercise through slow reps allow maximum time under tension with the loading applied against those muscle groups. Integrating new-school whole-body training and incorporating instability combine to heighten the muscle activity and peak contractions.

The program is composed of three supersets, each consisting of three exercises. Complete all three exercises in a superset before resting for 1 minute and then repeat for a total of three supersets. Once you have completed three rounds, rest for 2 full minutes before advancing to the next superset in your workout.

Exercise

Wrap sit-up: 3 × 15 slow

+ Barbell hip extension with medicine ball squeeze: 3 × 12 slow with pause at top

+ Squat to supine to sit-up: 3 × 10 each side with slow pause at top

Stability ball reverse rollout: 3 × 15 controlled tempo

+ Poor man's glute ham raise rollout: 3 × 12 controlled

+ Supine lower-abdominal cable curl: 3 × 10 slow with pause

Hanging knee raise with medicine ball: 3 × 15 controlled temp

+ Single-leg stride squat: 3 × 10 each side

Leg–hip–core multidirectional control: 3 × 12 each position

Body Reset

Program Description

This program focuses on maximizing full-body movement by enhancing mobility and flexibility. The loading is minimal but the movements itself are challenging. This is challenging not only physically but also mentally. You might feel uncomfortable as you attempt to regain lost mobility from either too much heavy lifting or too little exercise. After a thorough warm-up of 6 to 8 minutes of aerobic exercise of your choice and some dynamic movement, perform the following as combination sets. Rest 60 to 90 seconds between each set and exercise combination.

Exercise

Medicine ball squat-away: 3×10

Stability ball thoracic mobility: 3×8 to each side

Barbell hip extension with medicine ball squeeze: 3×10

Hip extension and knee flexion: 3×10

Prone row external rotation: 3×8

Prone medicine ball transfer: 3×8 each direction

Static lateral crunch with medicine ball punchout: 3×10 each side

Prone balance: 3×60 seconds

Strength

Program Description

The focus of this program is defined by its name, strength. It is the foundation for everything the body attempts to achieve in movement. In many group class formats strength is largely ignored in favor of explosive-type movements. All of these movements are meant to be slow and controlled. Do not use momentum to initiate the exercises. You should feel tension throughout the range of motion during the concentric and eccentric phase of each repetition. After a thorough warm-up, complete the following.

Exercise

Stability ball split squat with dumbbell: 3 × 8

Alternating stability ball hip extension with single-leg eccentric knee flexion: 3 × 8 to each side

Squat to ballast ball to Romanian deadlift: 3 × 6-8

Dip with medicine ball squeeze: 3 × 6-8

Supine pull-up: 3 × 8

Static split lunge to dumbbell lateral raise: 3 × 8 each direction

Supine pull-up: 3 × 8 each side

Strength ball decline dumbbell press: 3 × 6-8

▶ Muscle Up

Program Description

This program is for those who wish to pack on some muscle. Compared with the other programs, this program's combination exercises complement one other, through compounding, which involves hitting the same muscle group with two continuous exercises. This program is divided into lower-body and upper-body progressions. Complete each one twice per week. Try the lower body on Monday and Thursday, and the upper body on Tuesday and Friday.

Lower Body

Wall squat: 4×10

Stability ball split squat with dumbbell: 4×8

Poor man's glute ham raise rollout: $4 \times 8\text{-}10$

Hip extension and knee flexion: 4×12

Walking lunge with overhead medicine ball rotation: 3×10

Medicine ball split Russian twist: 3×10

Stability ball side-supported hip extension: 3×10

Standing bar twist with medicine ball squeeze: 3×8

Upper Body

Incline dumbbell press: 4×10

Supine pull-up: 4×10

Stability ball pull-up: $4 \times 8\text{-}10$

Pullover: 4×10

Prone front raise lateral fly: 3×10

Cross-body rear delt raise: 3×10

Stability ball reverse rollout: 3×10

Strong Kids

Program Description

One of the most common questions we receive has to do with kids: "When can my son or daughter start strength training?" There is so much misinformation in the public domain that it sometimes frightens parents. The research is strong on this topic and has studied kids as young as 7 years old. We do not typically start kids that young, but we do recommend that kids at those ages start with good fundamental sports like gymnastics and swimming, which promote all-around athleticism and are fun for young minds and bodies. In the gym environment, it's good to start at 12 years old with a progressive program focusing on fundamentals to ensure a solid development base as kids mature into full strength and conditioning programs.

Exercise

Medicine ball squat-away: 3 × 10

Reverse balance push-up (ball on thighs): × 8-10

Hip extension knee flexion: 3 × 10

Bridge T fall-off: 3 × 12

One-arm dumbbell press: 3 × 12

Supine lat pull and delt raise: 3 × 12

Abdominal side crunch: 3 × 10

Ax chop with hip flexion: 3 × 10

16-Week Program

In the 16-week program you are progressively introduced to the exercises described in the book. If you are just starting out, there will certainly be a temptation to jump ahead to some of the more difficult exercises, especially if you find some of the beginner-level exercises too easy. But stay on course. Take the time to build your foundation with the prescribed progressions, and your result will be a successful program. The time you put into the program in the first 4 to 6 weeks will ensure your success by helping you avoid soft-tissue injuries and reinforcing the techniques as described.

The exercises in the 16-week program provide an excellent array of strength, balance, and flexibility challenges. After the tables of most of the 4-week cycles are explanations of why specific combinations of exercises are used. After you have completed this program, you will be ready to design your own strength ball program.

Tempo and rest are two components that can dictate the direction of your program. The numbers in the tempo column are defined first. For example, 3:2:2 means that you lower the weight in 3 seconds, hold the middle position for 2 seconds, and raise the weight in 2 seconds. When a muscle causes a joint to move, it always results in shortening or lengthening of the working muscle. The first digit indicates lowering of the weight, which generally means you put a specific muscle through an eccentric contraction, or lengthening. The last digit indicates that you perform a concentric contraction, or shortening of the muscle.

The number in the rest column represents how much time you should take after a particular exercise. The exercises provide a number of supersets, where one exercise is followed immediately by a second exercise, then followed by a specific rest interval. This concept of supersetting is a means of making your workout efficient. Instead of working each muscle individually, you use an opposite muscle group (such as chest and upper back) or an upper-body and lower-body combination (such as chest and hamstrings). As you adapt to your program, you can apply the concept of progression to your rest periods to continually increase the intensity of your workouts. By attempting to shorten your rest time you will increase the metabolic intensity of the program, thereby imposing a greater challenge to your body and improving your endurance. You can also increase your rest time, especially if you want to lift very heavy loads. Increasing the rest time will provide you with greater recovery, which is an important component of high-level strength.

Weeks 1 to 4

Exercise	Sets × reps or time	Tempo	Rest period
1a. Wall squat	2-3 × 15-20	3:0:2	0
1b. Back extension	2-3 × 60 sec	Hold	2 min
2a. Single-leg hip lift	2-3 × 10	2:2:2	0
2b. Incline dumbbell press	2-3 × 15	3:0:2	1.5 min
3a. Pullover	2-3 × 12	3:2:2	0
3b. Hip extension and knee flexion	2-3 × 12	Slow	1.5 min
4a. McGill side raise with static hip adduction	2-3 × 30 sec	Hold	0
4b. Supine pull-up	2-3 × 12	3:1:2	1.5 min
5a. Prone balance	2-3 × 30-45 sec	Hold	0
5b. Bridge T fall-off	2-3 × 8-10 to each side	Slow	1.5 min

Finish with the following flexibility exercises, holding each position for 20 to 30 seconds for one or two sets:

1. Spinal extension
2. Lateral side stretch
3. Standing hamstring stretch
4. Standing lat and pec stretch
5. Kneeling posterior shoulder stretch

Note: In combos 1 and 5 we keep the grouping close together. Superset 1 focuses on legs and glutes in the wall squat and glutes, hamstrings, and spinal erectors in the back extension. This focus on the core and legs is a superset of the same muscle group to enhance hypertrophy and strength of this area. This is a foundation that you need to focus on for later progressions.

In superset 5 the focus is similar to the previous supersets except that we target the abdominals in a sagittal plane followed by a rotary stability challenge—same grouping, different planes.

Weeks 5 to 8

Exercise	Sets × reps or time	Tempo	Rest period
1a. Wall squat with weight	2-3 × 12-15	3:0:2	0
1b. Back extension	2-3 × 90-120 sec	Hold	2 min
2a. Hip extension and knee flexion	2-3 × 10	2:2:2	0
2b. One-arm dumbbell press	2-3 × 12	3:0:2	1.5 min
3a. One-arm pullover	2-3 × 12	3:2:2	0
3b. One-leg hip extension and knee flexion	2-3 × 12	Slow	1.5 min
4a. McGill side raise with static hip adduction	2-3 × 10-12	2:1:2	0
4b. Eccentric accentuated biceps curl	2-3 × 10	3:1:2	1.5 min
5a. Prone balance hip opener	2-3 × 10	Slow	0
5b. Bridge with medicine ball drops	2-3 × 10-12	Fast	1.5 min

Finish with the following flexibility exercises, holding each position for 20 to 30 seconds for one or two sets:

1. Spinal extension
2. Lateral side stretch
3. Standing hamstring stretch
4. Standing lat and pec stretch
5. Kneeling posterior shoulder stretch

Weeks 9 to 12

Exercise	Sets × reps or time	Tempo	Rest period
1a. Single-leg wall squat	2-3 × 6-8	2:0:2	0
1b. Reverse back extension	2-3 × 8-12	3:0:3	2 min
2a. One-leg hip extension and knee flexion	2-3 × 8-10	Slow	0
2b. Dual-ball fly	2-3 × 8-12	3:0:2	1.5 min
3a. Cross-body rear delt raise	2-3 × 10-12	3:2:2	0
3b. Prone row external rotation	2-3 × 10-12	3:1:2	1.5 min
4a. Kneeling hold and clock	2-3 × 30-60 sec	Hold	0
4b. Incline triceps extension	2-3 × 12	3:0:2	1.5 min
5a. Jackknife	2-3 × 10-15	2:2:2	0
5b. Twister	2-3 × 10-12	Slow	1.5 min

Finish with the following flexibility exercises, holding each position for 20 to 30 seconds for one or two sets:

1. Spinal extension
2. Lateral side stretch
3. Standing hamstring stretch
4. Standing lat and pec stretch
5. Kneeling posterior shoulder stretch

Note: As you progress into week 9, you increase the intensity through several methods. For the legs, progress to unilateral squats, which are significantly more difficult than bilateral movements for the legs. The movements are multidirectional and therefore harder to stabilize, and the loading on the legs also changes. We also superset a chest and hamstring exercise. Both are considered advanced level. This combination will significantly increase the metabolic challenge as well as the strength challenge.

Weeks 13 to 16

Exercise	Sets × reps or time	Tempo	Rest period
1a. Poor man's glute ham raise rollout	2-3 × 8-10	Slow	2 min
2a. Supine lat pull and delt raise	2-3 × 8-10	Slow	0
3a. Supine dumbbell press and fly	2-3 × 10-12	2:0:2	0
3b. Supine rotator scissors	2-3 × 10-12	2:0:2	1.5 min
4a. Wrap sit-up	2-3 × 12-15 sec	3:0:2	0
4b. Medicine ball push-up	2-3 × 12	2:0:2	1.5 min
5b. Goldy's static lateral helicopter	2-3 × 10-12	Slow	1.5 min

Finish with the following flexibility exercises, holding each position for 20 to 30 seconds for one or two sets:

1. Spinal extension
2. Lateral side stretch
3. Standing hamstring stretch
4. Standing lat and pec stretch
5. Kneeling posterior shoulder stretch

Note: In the final cycle the exercises progress to very advanced. Most notably we introduce the challenge of contralateral movements within the same exercise for the supine lat pull and delt raise, and we introduce the concept of working the same muscle but with different movements from one side to the other with the supine dumbbell press and fly.

REFERENCES

Anderson, K., and D.G. Behm. 2005. Trunk muscle activity increases with unstable squat movements. *Canadian Journal of Applied Physiology* 30(1):33-45.

Berg, K. 1989. Balance and its measure in the elderly: A review. *Physiotherapy* 41:240-246.

Chu, D. and G. Myer 2013. *Plyometrics*. Champaign, IL: Human Kinetics.

Fradkin, A., T.R. Zazryn, and J.M. Smoliga. 2010. Effects of warming-up on physical performance: A systematic review with meta-analysis. *Journal of Strength & Conditioning Research* 24 (1):140-148.

Kinakin, K. *Optimal muscle training*. 2008. Champaign, IL: Human Kinetics.

Lederman, E. 2010. The myth of core stability. *Journal of Bodywork and Movement Therapies* 14 (1):84-98.

Lephart, S., et al. 1997. The role of proprioception in the management and rehabilitation of athletic injuries. *American Journal of Sports Medicine* 25(1):130-137.

McGill, S. 2015. Low back exercises: Evidence for improving exercise regimes. *Physical Therapy* 78(7):754-765.

McGill, S. 2015. *Low back disorders*. 3rd ed. Champaign, IL: Human Kinetics.

Posner-Mayer, J. 1995. *Swiss ball applications for orthopedic and sports medicine*. Denver: Ball Dynamics International.

Richardson, C. et al. 1999. *Therapeutic exercise for spinal segmental stabilization in low back pain*. Edinburgh: Churchill Livingstone.

Wirhed, R. 1990. *Athletic ability and the anatomy of motion*. London: Wolfe.

Yan, C.F., Y.C. Hung, M.L. Gau, and K.C. Lin. 2014. Effects of a stability ball exercise programme on low back pain and daily life interference during pregnancy. *Midwifery* 30(4):412-9.

ABOUT THE AUTHORS

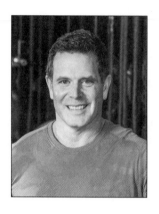

Lorne Goldenberg is the director of the UPMC Sports Performance Complex in Pittsburgh, Pennsylvania. The Sports Performance Complex provides services to athletes of all ages, skill levels, and sports along with nonathletes and others seeking to improve their fitness. He works with athletes in all sports, making them total-body strong and breaking new ground in targeted injury prevention, surgery, rehabilitation, training, and performance. Goldenberg is the former owner of the Athletic Conditioning Center and Strength Tek Fitness and Wellness Consultants, which provides service to more than 20,000 people throughout North America in Ottawa, Toronto, Montreal, and Boston.

Goldenberg has been active in the field of sport performance for over 30 years. Having worked in the National Hockey League (NHL) and Canadian Football League (CFL), he has served the Montreal Canadiens, Florida Panthers, Ottawa Senators, Ottawa Rough Riders, St. Louis Blues, Chicago Blackhawks, Quebec Nordiques, Colorado Avalanche, Windsor Spitfires, Owen Sound Attack, Ottawa 67's, and the University of Ottawa football team. Players such as Daniel Alfredsson, Daniel Briere, Zach Bogosian, Steven Stamkos, and Matt Bradley are just a few who seek out his expertise.

Goldenberg graduated from the University of Ottawa with an honors degree in physical education and is certified by the National Strength and Conditioning Association as a strength and conditioning specialist. He is also a certified exercise physiologist (CEP) through the Canadian Society for Exercise Physiology.

Goldenberg has published numerous articles in journals and magazines, including Men's Journal, Physical, and Ironman. As a conference presenter, he has established himself as one of the key sources for the major fitness and health conferences in North America. He has presented for organizations such as the National Strength and Conditioning Coaches Association, IDEA Health & Fitness Association, CanFitPro, American Fitness Professionals & Associates, Perform Better, Twist Conditioning, Yale University, and Dalhousie University.

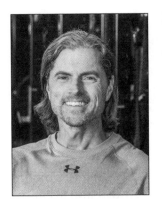

Peter Twist is the president and CEO of Twist Conditioning, an athlete conditioning company with franchised centers in the United States and Canada. His company offers one-on-one and team training, a line of 350 sport fitness products, and sport conditioning specialist certifications delivered by Twist master coaches throughout Canada, the United States, Australia, and the United Kingdom. A frequent guest lecturer at international fitness conferences and coaching clinics, Twist delivers workshops on sport conditioning to personal trainers, conditioning coaches, sport coaches, teachers, and medical professionals.

Twist has coached more than 700 professional athletes, including Hakeem Olajuwon, Mark Messier, and Justin Morneau, and was the NHL conditioning coach and exercise physiologist for the Vancouver Canucks (Stanley Cup finalists 1994) for 11 years. An NSCA-certified strength and conditioning specialist and CanFitPro personal training specialist with a master's degree in coaching science from the University of British Columbia, Twist served as president of the Hockey Conditioning Coaches Association, editor of the Journal of Hockey Conditioning, and NSCA provincial director for British Columbia.

Twist has authored 10 books, 16 DVDs, and more than 400 articles on sport-specific conditioning. A previous honoree of the CanFitPro Specialty Presenter of the Year and recipient of the Business Excellence Award as Business Person of the Year, Twist was the 2013 IDEA World Fitness Inspiration Award honoree for his leading example of living life to its fullest.

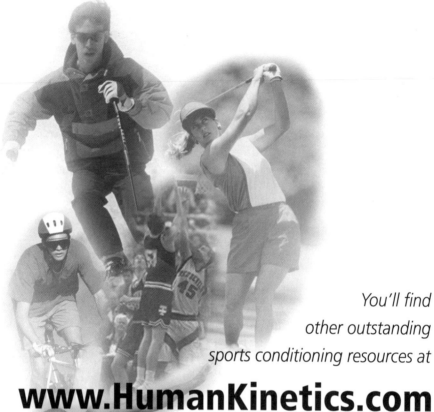

*You'll find
other outstanding
sports conditioning resources at*

www.HumanKinetics.com

In the U.S. call

1-800-747-4457

Australia............................. 08 8372 0999
Canada 1-800-465-7301
Europe......................+44 (0) 113 255 5665
New Zealand........................ 0800 222 062

HUMAN KINETICS
The Premier Publisher for Sports & Fitness
P.O. Box 5076 • Champaign, IL 61825-5076 USA